T0383501

Swimming
with the
Viking of Skye

For W.D., who taught me about courage.

Swimming
with the
Viking of Skye

A true story of overcoming fear
and finding hope for the future

RICHARD WATERS

Aurum

Acknowledgements

Thanks to my friend Matt Rhodes for his noble spirit and patience, my children Finn and Agatha, and my sister Loubie. To my parents for their unflagging support, and the brilliant team at Aurum who always believed in this book when at times its completion hung in the balance due to my health; special thanks to Richard Green. And finally, my gratitude to the magical Isle of Skye, without whose freezing lochs and waterfalls this book might never have happened.

Quarto

First published in hardback in 2025 by Aurum,
an imprint of Quarto
One Triptych Place,
London, SE1 9SH
United Kingdom
www.Quarto.com/Aurum

EEA Representation, WTS Tax d.o.o.,
Žanova ulica 3, 4000 Kranj, Slovenia

A catalogue record for this book is
available from the British Library.

ISBN: 978-0-7112-9189-8
Ebook ISBN: 978-0-7112-9191-1
Audiobook ISBN: 978-0-7112-9617-6

2 4 6 8 10 9 7 5 3 1

Map by Martin Brown
Typeset in Bembo Infant MT by seagulls.net
Printed and bound by CPI Group (UK) Ltd, Croydon, CR0 4YY

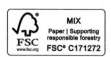

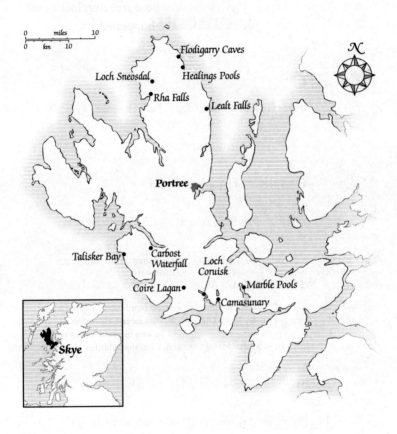

miles 0 — 10

km 0 — 10

N

Flodigarry Caves

Loch Sneosdal

Healings Pools

Rha Falls

Lealt Falls

Portree

Carbost
Waterfall

Talisker Bay

Loch
Coruisk

Coire Lagan

Marble Pools

Camasunary

Skye

Contents

Foreword

Every now and then we all meet someone who, without realising, makes our life that little bit brighter. Having come to know Richard through writing two of my own books (Richard being my editor), it's safe to say he left me with a lasting impression and I hoped that we would remain friends. When he asked me to write the Foreword for his book, not only did I know a strong friendship had been forged but I felt proud and honoured to do so.

Richard is one of life's rarities; he emanates a warmth and calmness few possess. Somehow, whenever we talk, whether he knows it or not, I always come away feeling that it's all going to be okay. It was only while reading this book that I began to understand why Richard has these qualities.

Richard's life tapestry has often been woven with serious misfortune and hardship. Diagnosed with Parkinson's at such a young age, only to then discover that his three-year-old daughter had a degenerative illness that would render her unable to talk or walk, turned his entire world upside down and has set him on a soul-searching journey ever since. His diagnosis alone is enough to break many but to find out your own child is destined to suffer in such a way and have absolutely no control over it is every parent's greatest fear – enough to send anyone on a downward spiral.

This is where Richard's story comes into its own. Not only does he write so honestly and openly about his struggles and the battles deep within himself, but Richard's determination to not succumb to his illness or any of life's other pressures leads him to embark on a powerful journey of self-discovery and a search for inner peace.

Swimming with the Viking of Skye is a beautiful tale of how a person can use the healing powers of Mother Nature and wild swimming as a way to reconnect with themselves. As an adventurer myself, who lived for six years in the great outdoors and the wilds of Scotland, I understand this power more than most. Similarly to Richard, my immersion into the wild stripped away all the white noise surrounding me.

Richard perfectly explains his relationship with nature and how it helped him to edge away from the clutter of modern-day life, lay to rest his regrets and focus the mind and body on what's really important in life: self-fulfilment.

While reading this book, I found myself reflecting deeply on the philosophy of life Richard draws upon and it reminded me of the importance of having clarity in my life as well as a strong sense of focus and self-worth. Richard is true to himself, kind and compassionate, and shows us the importance of never lying down on your belly and being tickled by what we can't control. I'd challenge anyone who doesn't feel the urge to wild swim after reading this – a beautifully written book full of life lessons by an inspiring human being, my friend, Richard.

Christian Lewis

Introduction

It's often said that we should count our blessings in life, look to the things which make us happy and be grateful for them. For me, gratitude is the key foundation to achieving positive personal transformation and recognising the gifts in your everyday, like your partner, your children, your friends and the food on your plate. Saying thank you for the things you already have tells you that you are doing okay, and it instantly changes the way you are feeling and turns your face to the sunshine rather than keeping you focused on the things you lack, or all the things that are going wrong for you. Telling yourself you will only be really happy when you've attained something or solved a current worry, hangs all your energy on an external something, whereas a richer inner life, being happy from within, is what will truly bring you fulfilment.

It was 2011, and I had a lot to be grateful for. My children Finn and Agatha, whom I was so proud of, were both healthy. They were also funny, kind and imaginative individuals and – most importantly – good friends to one another. I couldn't have asked for more. Finn, the elder of the two, was seven years old at the time this story starts; fun-loving, creative and fiercely protective of his sister. Aggie was three years old, possessed of a determination, a wicked sense of fun and arrestingly beautiful. As a baby she looked like a cherub in a kid's illustrated book. My ex-wife Ali was and still is a strong, effervescent woman with a big heart who can light up a room as she enters it. Not only does she have a strong presence, but she draws people towards her with her laugh and earthiness. My older sister Lou and I have always understood each other, and been the best of friends. I was close to my parents. I also had a strong base of male friendships, some of which had been forged twenty years earlier at school, as well as a couple of trusted girlfriends. So, I had a lot to be grateful for.

Principally, I was a travel author and wrote books for Lonely Planet. I was also a freelance travel journalist for broadsheets like the *Telegraph* and the *Sunday Times*, and glossy magazines such as *Elle*. I often worked for businesses, training individuals to deal with difficult personalities in awkward situations. It was a mix of role-play acting and psychology, a skill set left over from my days as an actor.

I have always measured my wealth by the richness of my experiences rather than noughts on a balance sheet, and unconsciously, I suppose, I designed my life to be one of contrasts. I considered myself blessed to be able to take my family on some amazing trips, the first of which was to Bern in Switzerland, where our hotel overlooked the peaks of the Bernese Oberland, and we stayed in a suite that had served as a temporary home to John le Carré and Fidel Castro (not at the same time, although that would have made for an interesting book!).

Solo travel assignments took me all over the world, and although I was there to work, I am still grateful to my wife for giving me the latitude to be able to disappear off for weeks or sometimes a month. In Laos, I shared the back seat of a decrepit bus with Hmong tribeswomen and cages of bats. In Puerto Vallarta, I stayed at Richard Burton's beautiful old Mexican hacienda where he lived with Suzy Hunt after she divorced the racing driver James Hunt, and he divorced Elizabeth Taylor. I witnessed wild orangutans in Kalimantan; swam with giant turtles in the cerulean waters of the Celebes Sea; heard the howl of wolves in the Carpathian Mountains; and tracked the world's largest bears on Kodiak Island, Alaska. I had looked for great whites in Martha's Vineyard, and even free-dived with sperm whales in the Caribbean Windward Islands. In short, I had been on adventures and enjoyed access to fascinating people and storied places money alone cannot buy. My father used to say I had lived the lives of many men combined. Up until wrecking ball number one ripped into my healthy body and introduced a dark interloper called 'progressive illness', things were really good. But like most of us, I took it all for granted.

Although my relationship with water has been a close one throughout my life, it's only since becoming a wild

swimmer that I have learnt just how life-giving and nourishing this vital element is. I was a champion swimmer
as a teenager, and unbeaten, I broke longstanding school
records. Short-lived competitive wins in a pool full of
chlorine might make for pleasant memories for the ego,
but there is no comparison to that immediate sense of
having tasted nature's soul tonic, which is what the freezing embrace of natural wild water inspires. All my teenage
triumphs in the pool essentially roll into a single memory
of winning, yet I can pretty much remember all my cold
swims separately, or at least the ones on Skye.

Within these pages, I describe some of the mental
approaches I developed to find happiness within that dark
province called degenerative illness. The thing about any
health condition which is progressive is that since it gets
worse over a period of time and irrevocably, you had
better arm yourself with some mental processes to deal
with it. Every cloud has a silver lining and the benefits of
having a long-term illness that is gradually going to get
worse is that you have more time to *gradually* prepare for it.
But if you don't try out different ways of thinking that can
help you, you're not going to get past the first year or two;
the illness will take you over, chew you up in its maw and
spit you out. I want to share the pillars I used to support
the roof of my sanity, in case they prove useful in whatever
you might be going through. It is often said that we only
grow in moments of adversity, when events shake us to the
core and turn our lives upside down; when circumstances

are so difficult it can feel as if we're being tested in a kind of celestial endurance game. What was that line in King Lear? 'As flies to wanton boys are we to the gods, they kill us for their sport.' Well, the times I'll tell you about were sometimes *beyond* difficult and I learnt a fair bit about myself. In particular, that humans are capable of shouldering an awful lot. We are much tougher than we realise.

I believe there is comfort in recognising that nothing is forever, whether the bright times of equilibrium or when everything seems pitted against us. In life's flux, nothing is ever still: planets rotate, seasons change, and people we love move in and out of our lives beyond our control – some taken by illness, others by circumstance. Everything that we delight in must eventually be returned, be it riches, our favourite people, possessions or gardens and pets; we have them temporarily and then only on trust. And no matter how old you are, in the playground of life death is constantly playing 'What's the time Mr Wolf?' with you. So far, nobody has beaten it. But if we can submit to the universal truth that all of us are also in flux and we learn to roll with it, our days will be happier and freer.

Over the following pages you'll read where this illness took me and what I did to try and make sense of the unfolding mess, often unsuccessfully, and sometimes damaging others close to me in the process. We do desperate self-destructive things when we sense our end coming, when we are broken, and sometimes we find comfort in things we never expected to; like the ancient philosophy of Stoicism and wild swimming, both of which have saved my bacon. I can honestly say that if I hadn't experienced either of them, I would not be here writing this. On my spiritual journey, I certainly became more aware of my inner self through soul-searching, reading and trying to find meaning where at times it seemed there was none. And wild swimming took a charge of me like a benign sergeant, marching me to the water's edge again and again. This is my story.

Richard Waters

2024

Chapter 1

Double Diagnosis

In 2011, we – my wife, Ali, our kids, Finn and Agatha, and I – moved from Brighton to Cirencester in the Cotswolds. That's when this story begins. Of course, we instantly missed the sea and the liveliness of the city, standing in the queue for bagels behind Nick Cave (for noodles, it's Kevin Rowland), but had decided we wanted the kids to grow up in a more rural environment. Unintentionally, I seem to spend twelve years in each place that I've lived: just as for London, Brighton, for all its charms, was to be no exception. In Cirencester, we rented a charming but overpriced old cottage whilst we looked for a house to buy, which Ali could then transform with her interior design skills.

A few months later, I was in the French Alps on assignment for a broadsheet to do a travel piece on 'Learning to snowboard at 40'. By the time I got around to researching it, I was forty-one. It should have been great fun as most of my surfing buddies were going too; I think there were eight of us in total. The last time I'd tried snowboarding was twenty years earlier and then I had taken to it quite well, slaloming down black runs by the end of my first week. But this time, ye gods, I was *utter* crap, and I'm not being faux modest. I had no sense of balance whatsoever and kept falling over. My pals were veteran boarders, and being a beginner – at least until my current skill level drastically improved – I insisted they go off-piste, do their thing and not wait for me, while I quietly went about trying to re-nail this graceful sport. Strangely, I was also tired, so knackered that I could barely find the energy to walk back to the chalet in my hard bindings. And the fabled 'fear', when your body goes into flight mode – and not a sensation I was usually intimate with – had taken hold towards the end of the first day as I looked down from the top of a glittering red run of packed ice. I felt my whole body shaking, my battered coccyx already black and blue with bruising.

Falling down on ice patches was something I became adept at, and on the last day I really outdid myself when I tumbled backwards on ice heading down a steep incline, broke a back rib, slightly perforating a lung, and was stretchered down the mountain. That wasn't quite the denouement I ended the article with, but then nobody wants to read that taking up snowboarding again after twenty years' absence is a bad idea.

'Maybe you were just really tired, that's why you kept falling,' said my wife evenly, after she had picked me up at the airport, helped me hobble to the car and I was back home. 'You've been on the go for months.'

I'd been travelling a fair bit with work, and my level of weariness was off the chart; it made me want to lie down and nod off to sleep wherever I happened to be, like River Phoenix's character in *My Own Private Idaho*. And while I didn't have narcolepsy, something definitely wasn't right in the state of Denmark. There were other physical developments I noted; I had started typing words backwards and, if it was at all possible, I was being even more disorganised and forgetful than usual.

Ignorance is definitely bliss, and for the time being I managed to put these concerns in a box and denied them any more headspace. Amazing how you can have a demon growing in your back yard to which you are blithely oblivious. It was now May 2011, and I was on a travel assignment on Patmos, the Greek island where two thousand years ago, the disciple John the Divine experienced the hellish visions in a mountain cave that would later be transcribed as the Book of Revelation. One morning by the harbour, I, too, had my own rather less dramatic revelation when I noticed my right thumb involuntarily shaking. I had boxed throughout my thirties and had taken my fair share of knocks to the head, but no more than anyone else. And yes, there was a period when I was regularly concussed; I used to affectionately refer to that feeling of cranial numbness as 'sponge head'.

But it was not as if I had scores of fights notched up. I'd sparred with over twenty boxers over the years: some tough, gifted, fleetfooted and artful; others ponderous, flat-footed and two dimensional. My less-than-illustrious time in the ring had spanned about six years in total, of which around four were regularly spent sparring. I was sure 'the sweet science' was not responsible for the tremor I had developed in my right hand. 'Besides,' I arrogantly reminded myself, 'You're only forty-one!'

Still, that involuntary shaking of my thumb worried me and it was now getting more regular, more insistent. Ali would sometimes say, 'You were morse coding on my back last night,' meaning that I had been tapping away with my thumb or finger while I was fast asleep. And on top of the chronic fatigue, lack of balance and periodical mild tremoring, my sex life, which had always been a source of pleasure for Ali and I, and something we could reset our relationship's factory settings with, also came under attack as I started to experience ED and premature ejaculation. One night, I said to my wife, 'I think I better go and see a doctor ...'

It's a bit sad that it took for my sex life to be interrupted before I was sufficiently spooked to go and see my GP that same week, who then immediately referred me to a neurologist. A few weeks later, I learnt that all these new developments – lack of balance, sexual dysfunction, vivid dreams, mental confusion, typing backwards, chronic fatigue and increasing palsy – were all symptoms of 'Early Onset Parkinson's Disease'. The diagnosis was economically delivered by a doctor in a white room on a fine late summer's day in Cheltenham. Having delivered his bombshell, he seemed baffled, disappointed even, by my calm acceptance. 'You don't seem too perturbed by the diagnosis Mr Waters.'

'It is what it is,' I said flatly. 'I've got young children to feed and a roof to keep over their heads whether I am ill or not, so I'll just have to get on with it.'

He regarded me through thick myopic glasses and blinked, reminding me rather of a terrapin, 'Well, yes … that's very stoic of you,' he tailed off.

Actually, I was staggered by the revelation; I thought only old folk developed Parkinson's, not people my age. At forty-one, I was still a spring chicken. And when, a few days later, an official letter arrived from the hospital confirming my diagnosis, I read it, screwed it up and stuck it in the bin. Was I putting my head in the sand? Yes, but there was method in my madness. The demon in my back yard was now running amok, and if I accidentally fed him with fears of the future, he grew instantly bigger and frightened me. So I would starve him.

To this end, I wanted to know as little about the disease as possible. Then at least I wouldn't be aware of the forty-odd possible symptoms that might or might not be waiting for me further down the road of decline. Everybody's Parkinson's is slightly different: so while one person might experience extreme shaking, another might have a mild palsy but more pronounced dyskinesia, which produces involuntary movements of the body that gradually become more dramatic and exhausting. Ironically, dyskinesia develops as a side effect to the many meds you have to take to remain still. Looking back, I am still glad that I took the decision to go at it blind, and at this early stage the disease was entirely tolerable.

Up until the diagnosis it had been just a question of a shaking hand and severe fatigue, plus a few other things. The sexual problems, at least, had gone away, and I was still fulfilling my deadlines with the travel publisher. Only now, each book was taking a lot longer, with all the mistakes that needed correcting along the way, and all the jumbled up words. But it was manageable, so why catastrophise and make it any worse?

Because it is going to get worse.

Well, I'll worry about that when it does. In the meantime, I still have a living to earn.

Globally, there are around 9.4 million people living with Parkinson's Disease (PD). Over the past twenty-five years its prevalence has more than doubled. It is characterised by resting tremor, stiffness of limbs and bradykinesia (slowness of movement), as well as dyskinesia, which can be hugely exhausting. These are just the motor systems, however, and there's a rich list of non-motor symptoms, including depression, loss of taste and smell, mood changes, drooling, apathy, constipation and sleep problems.

Unless you're a complete lone wolf, I believe the following saying is true, 'The results you get in your life are in direct correlation to the standards your peer group holds you to.' In other words, we are a reflection of the views and people we surround ourselves with, and – depending on their opinions – our own convictions can either be strengthened or diluted by them. Our focus becomes so much narrower in our autumn years. Why is this the case? I think it's because when we stop working, or travel less, our immediate social circle becomes smaller, the people in it less diverse. Despite this, and in spite of the PD, I believed I was still a fighter, a young*ish* person who had so much more to do with his life, both for the sake of his kids and his own identity. I wasn't ready to give up and allow this disease to prematurely put me out to pasture, nor could I afford to allow that to happen.

Like a skilled Cuban featherweight boxer, PD comes at you slyly from all different angles, peppering you with jabs to the body and right hand crosses, slowly assailing you with the shakes (palsy), dyskinesia (or as Michael J. Fox puts it 'body dipping' like Axl Rose) and dystonia (the painful bunching of the fingers and toes), never mind losing your sense of smell. It's the decathlete of diseases, only it doesn't stop at ten special disciplines; there are thirty other symptoms, from hallucinations and rage, to loss of balance and falling over; freezing in midstride, stiffening of the limbs, dangerously deep depression and hot flushes, and an increase in impulsivity whereby you lose the ability to control gambling or sexual urges that previously would have been easily subdued. These are all delights PD gradually throws in to the mix to further derail you and those closest to you; it's the disease that keeps on giving!

Until your health is decimated by serious illness, you secretly think you're untouchable. Go on, admit it, there are those of you reading who'll be thinking: 'Bloody hell I'm lucky I've made it to sixty and so far, so good!' I say good luck to you, because up until 29 September 2011 I did, too. I had taken plenty of physical risks throughout my life – in the boxing ring, with wild animals and in restive, politically unstable countries where I'd worked as a writer – so why should I have the monopoly on being imperishable? Maybe I deserved it for pushing the envelope as far as I had, and doubtless, whichever guardian angel had been looking after me, was now clearly exhausted and had passed on the baton, but it seemed nobody else was up for it. I had taken my health for granted and never thought something like Parky would slip into my fortress like a coward through an open window and sink its claws into me.

I'd had barely a year to try and get my head around this unwanted intruder in my body when, towards the end of November 2012, yet another wrecking ball blindsided my wife and I. But it was a much fiercer blow, as we were told that Agatha, our beloved three-year-old daughter, had developed a degenerative neurological disorder, but one that hadn't yet been diagnosed The worst thing was that the medical establishment had not come across it before. In the presciently named Battledown Ward at Cheltenham Hospital, the kindly paediatrician delivered the news that it wasn't anything as harmless as 'glue-ear' or 'hypermobility' which we had hoped was causing our beautiful little girl to keep falling over, but that it was actually her brain under attack. Something sinister was making it produce too much protein, and it was that protein which was attacking her perfectly healthy neurons, as well as laying siege to something called the cerebellum. Sometimes called the 'little brain', it is massively important as it is responsible for balance and coordination, as well as helping with the development of speech.

Aggie's cerebellum was shrinking. 'Atrophy' was the cold and surgical name they used. The doctors and brain specialists just didn't know what was causing her brain to make the extra protein, and therefore had no idea how to treat it.

Presently, one female doctor illustrated this by pointing at a brain scan Aggie had had taken at Bristol Hospital two months earlier. Previously, she'd suggested Agatha have one 'just to be safe, to rule out anything unpleasant'. Watching Agatha wheeled unconscious into the MRI scanning room, her tiny little body and kid-size shoes taking up a fraction of the room available on the gurney, and the oxygen mask over her unformed face, it felt so wrong, I had never suspected life could be so cruel.

And so, here we were a few weeks after that scan in Battledown Ward, the doctor quietly and compassionately indicating gatherings of 'white matter' or 'protein' on the brain scan, and that accursed sentence 'atrophy of the cerebellum' was introduced to our vocabulary for the first time. It felt as if we were running out of time. I knew nothing about the cerebellum but I understood the meaning of the word 'atrophy'. It means to gradually waste away, to get weaker.

The doctor left us in peace for a few minutes to absorb the news, and before the door had shut both my wife and I had started to sob uncontrollably in each other's arms. It was a grief I had never experienced before. Looking back, whatever positive spin I might try to put on it, our life changed that day and it has never been the same since.

We were no longer in 'just to be sure there's nothing unpleasant' territory. No, now we had joined the tragic ranks of those whose boat has not glided over, but instead been snagged by, the reef of misfortune. It was hard not to feel that our family had been carefully selected to be tested and toyed with in a maze beyond the realm of fair play, far beyond what ordinary people are capable of dealing with. *As flies to wanton boys* ... the gods were having a fucking laugh, slowly ripping our wings off one at a time.

In comparison with Aggie's unnamed enemy, in its first couple of years my Parkinson's remained inoffensive and I just got on with things. It seemed a lot of the time my wife and I were waiting impatiently for more tests to be done on Aggie and hoping for some kind of progress for our little girl in the realm of getting a diagnosis and finding a cure. But how can you beat something that hasn't been identified? We felt absolutely powerless and at the mercy of neurologists who might or might not raise the issue at their next conference in the hope that other neurologists might keep an eye out for the condition and its symptoms. That's how far beyond Pluto we were. It felt as if we were at the edge of a lonely universe: there was nobody we could talk to, nobody else who'd been there and no one who understood what we were going through.

It is far better to know your enemy, to be able to size them up and figure out what their weak spots are, to learn from a tried and tested canon of knowledge based on how others before you have managed. There was still no cure for Parkinson's, but at least there was medication to bring it under control in its early days, and there was also the last stop café of deep brain stimulation – having your skull or chest prized open to receive a device which stopped the tremors by sending an electrical pulse to the specific part of the brain which caused the tremor. That was a long way away, presented serious risks and was reserved only for desperate measures. But with Aggie's illness, we were pitted against an invisible opponent in the dark: we didn't stand a chance as it developed quickly and began to rob her of basic things the rest of us take for granted, like balance.

The house we bought in 2012 needed an awful lot of work doing to it, as it had previously been a student house, but both my wife and I could see beyond the fag-burned carpets, jaundiced puke-yellow flocked walls and multiple toilets. It was an old Victorian redbrick, one of four villas with a New Orleans-style balcony out front. It was a huge space and radiated right back from the main road on which it sat. I would strip the floors and treat them, then we'd knock a few walls down and open the rooms up, and in no time it would become a cosy bolthole. An immediate problem, though, was the steep staircase, as one horrible morning Aggie lost her balance and fell down it, literally head over heels. I was downstairs, halfway into the living room, so I could only watch. I had to pick her up off the floor on which she lay spreadeagled, facedown, and I felt her anguish and surprise. As I held her close to me and tried to quieten her sobs, I felt her heart hammering with shock. Needless to say, we put a gate across the passageway at the top of the stairs to ward of any repeat falls. I was so angry with life.

What was utterly mind-boggling was that there was no previous timeline of another person who had suffered her illness – as there was no name for it – so we had no idea how long she had to live and whether it was possible to find a cure in the remaining time. One doctor uselessly suggested it was better just to love her as much as we could and not bother dragging her to various pointless appointments with specialists who really didn't know what was going on in her brain. Then, unconsciously, she turned the tap on beside her and proceeded to wash her hands. Just as we had put up a stairgate, we now built a wall around us as protection from what felt like the medical establishment's defeatism. Ali and I decided that we would take matters into our own hands and try complementary medicine rather than waiting for conventional science to produce a cure. My sister Lou is one of life's pure souls and as long as I can remember she has been a healer, be it of animals or people. She is also a qualified homeopath and urged me to try this medicine. The basis of homeopathy, she explained, was treating like with like, and that we all have a vital force within us that maintains a balance in our health. When this force becomes unsettled, we fall ill. I thought I'd try it out on myself first before Aggie had a go.

I went to see a homeopath in Swansea a week before I was due to drive a cheap hire car – literally a hairdryer with wheels – thousands of miles around Romania for a month with travel work. The homeopath prescribed me something that really helped stop my tremors. I don't know whether *it* was doing the work or whether the prescription was a placebo and it was me, but when, halfway through Transylvania I broke the bottle accidentally, the shakes soon returned.

In early 2013, Ali and I took Aggie to see the homeopath in Cardiff, who prescribed her a remedy called Nux Vom. Within minutes of leaving the homeopath's office, her vital force seemed to rally and Aggie was like a mustang that just wanted to gallop. There was no stopping her; we just had to make sure we held on to her so she didn't fall over. The tablet worked for a while, but after a few days we were back to square one.

Agatha has never ever complained or asked why she can no longer walk, no longer feed herself, why she needs to be carried to the loo, and why she can't speak. But I know our girl must have compared herself to others and wondered why, unlike her, they never fell over and why she was constantly losing her balance. She has the most beautiful soul.

I remember my eyes filling as Aggie's nursery school teacher told my wife and I how sufficiently self-aware our girl was that she stepped to one side when it was 'garden time' so as to let all the boys rush past her, before she walked at her own pace precariously on to the grass outside. She knew she was different, that she wasn't as quick in her speech or movements as her peers, and with grace and dignity she was doing the best a three-year-old could to navigate the difficulties she was dealing with.

Our girl looks like a younger version of Julie Christie, she is drop-dead gorgeous. I remember all those conversations we went on to have with her teachers as we fretted about how she was going to manage in the nativity play or whatever performance they were putting on. From free-standing while singing – but usually hidden at the back, close to the teacher's assistant (who could catch her if she fell) – to eventually being seated on a bench (at the back), then in a wheelchair, her physical decline was watched in slow motion by sympathetic parents in the audience, all of whom I'm sure at one point quietly thanked their God he had spared their children such an ordeal.

The medical establishment were right about Aggie's decline; in the first years it came steady and stealthy. All the while her coordination and motor skills diminished: first she was unable to balance; then she could no longer walk; then she lost the ability to talk, something she had done little of anyway. Each of these milestones of deterioration impacted massively on her quality of life; she couldn't paint, play with dolls, ride a bike, nor could we leave her with a friend unless she was within sight in case she fell over.

Not to be beaten, for a while Aggs hopped and pulled her way up to the summit of our three-storeyed Victorian house. As of 2016, I watched Aggie slide into the maw of an illness, which took so much from her with such rabidity, that I began to lose my mojo. In the first five years of my illness, from 2011 to 2016, my own health, too, had begun to deteriorate noticeably, with worsening shakes and near-constant fatigue.

Though I tried to keep both of these hidden, I was also beginning to experience depression, which would do its best to make me wallow in self-pity. I tried my best to cast it off, sought to look for the good things in each day that I had to be grateful for to counter the black thoughts in my head. But the pain of what was happening to Aggie was just too raw to bear. Ali was obviously devastated by what was happening to our little girl, and the way she dealt with it was to pour all her energies into Agatha and her new business.

Ali had started the business with one of the mums at school back in 2012. It was the age of shabby chic and they were painting up and distressing old cupboards and furniture to sell in the local arts market.

I'd taken Aggie's little bike to the bike shop where they fitted extra-large pedals with straps on top of them to hold her feet in place, but when we tried something as straight-forward as having her complete a single revolution of the pedal, something short-circuited in her brain, stopped it from happening and her legs would jar.

We took Aggie to a physio every week to keep our girl's now inactive legs from seizing up, and to treat her 'dystonia', the involuntary muscle contractions that caused her legs to twist, and her toes and fingers to bunch pain-fully. The muscles soon atrophied in her once chunky legs, and despite using the stairs as a means of building up her thighs and calves – all the while repeating the mantra 'use it or lose it', referring to her legs – the energy it required from her made it impossible to climb them.

Our family was not complete without Finn, our first-born, son and my best friend. When he was still in Ali's womb, I played him the instrumental music of Brian Eno with the speaker next to Ali's tummy. After he was born, if he was ever upset, we only had to play either of Eno's two ambient songs, 'An Ending' or 'Deep Blue Day' to reassure him and he would abruptly stop crying, and smile. It worked a treat; on some pre-congenital level he must have remembered the soothing music and safety of his mother's womb. He still loves it to this day and is heavily influenced by music throughout his work in film and photography.

As Finn was growing up, every night when I was home, I read him stories about the Greek myths. I introduced him to the multiverse of Marvel superheroes, taught him how to box and have an inner moral code to stick up for others weaker than himself. After we moved from Brighton to the Cotswolds when he was about six and I was forty years old, he kept his head down in his new school and fitted in quickly with the children around him. I was so proud of him for the way he made that tricky adjustment. Finn was a bright ray of boyishness who was at his happiest drawing, being in the company of friends or playing with his little sister. Sometimes, we would write stories together about ghosts and werewolves; he certainly inherited my love of the gothic and seeking out adventure. He was, and still is, very much a free spirit, and would disappear with his friends on their bikes for long summer days looking at deserted buildings.

We had been in the Cotswolds no more than a month when I took an assignment in Borneo to update and rewrite a huge section of the country for the Lonely Planet travel guide to Kalimantan, the wildest and least mapped area.

Ironically, for somebody who loved travelling, I didn't possess the necessary characteristics of the perfect travel writer. I got homesick: I only had to think of my children and the amount of time we would be separated, and, whether I was bouncing along on a bus in dark mountains or on a night flight in an old prop plane, it would bring a tear to my eyes. When I was starting out travel writing, a few years before our move to the Cotswolds, a seasoned hack and friend assured me that I would soon get used to not seeing my kids, and that homesickness was just a switch in my mind that I would learn to flick off. He couldn't have been more wrong.

Fresh from the Bornean jungles, and relieved to be back in Cirencester, I had the dirt of an ex-cannibal village still in my fingernails. Here, I had seen a local boy's head split open like a watermelon after his bike slid off one of the narrow mountain paths and he fell a great height. A slow rumble of drums issued from a hut, where the shaman was doing his best to administrate magic to the boy who lay dying on his floor. Half the village was packed in. Just in case his chicken bones didn't work, the witch doctor had placed a packet of Anadin close to the boy's head. He was dead by the morning. Death could come to us at any time just like it had to this boy; the difference is in the West we don't expect to die until we develop a terminal disease, whereas in the developing world it is a given that death is never far away. I needed to live more appreciatively, making the most of the time I had.

On this trip I'd felt so far away from my children and wife, so powerless to stop both my daughter's and my own disease in their tracks. I had also noted that I found the humidity intolerable and that everything felt heavier, and everywhere seemed longer to walk. I responded by giving myself more time to do things rather than trying to keep going at my previous rate.

Now home, I was crestfallen that little Aggs was no surer on her feet. What was I expecting to have happened in my absence? A miracle? My spirit settled back into gloom mode. I was returning to what felt like a terrible dream. I now had four gears: depressed, anxious, angry and fearful (in no particular order). I was afraid. I didn't know how rapidly this disease would evolve for Aggie and I knew little about the one I was suffering from myself. Fear often masks itself behind anger; if I questioned the merits of the universe that it had given me Parkinson's, I was fucking furious and hated it doubly for what it had thrown at my daughter. I had four years of hard sparring which might explain why I had developed Parky; however little Aggs had done *nothing* to invite this.

My wife and I would sometimes look at each other, shake our heads and say, 'This is a joke, does anyone we know have such bad luck as us?' Or, 'We are going to wake up one morning and say, "Phew, thank God, it was just a bad nightmare, nothing is that bad!"'

I felt like I was running down, like a kind of toy that needs winding up. My spatial awareness was increasingly becoming shot to bits, and I began to walk into doorjambs or bump into people in shops. Water had always been my sanctuary but when I went to the local pool to swim laps – which I usually did three times a week – I found that just to hit thirty laps was taking forever, and my front-crawl, which had been clean and fluid, was now unco-ordinated and sloppy because of my right arm dragging.

By the time Christmas 2012 arrived, I'd hired an office in town to have somewhere quiet where I could focus and write up the Borneo book quickly. A few nights before Christmas Eve I was alone in the old building where I kept an office. The wooden floorboards beneath the threadbare carpets were warped with age, and creaked as you walked upon them, while the walls were open beamed and dated back to Elizabethan times. My room sat directly above the WH Smith which was on the ground floor below. The heating was turned off and tubes of steam shot from my mouth as I worked, my Arctic coat keeping me warm. The staff of the estate agent's I shared the space with had gone home for the night; it was just me. Through the mullioned windows I could see the snow falling softly on the crooked roofs of Cirencester.

When I went to the loo across the corridor that night I felt as if someone on the landing was watching me. It wasn't a pleasant feeling. Feeling uneasy, I wrapped up writing for the night, saved my progress on my laptop and put my notes away in my briefcase. Then I locked the door to my office and turned out the light in the corridor, finding my way down the stairs in the darkness. The feeling of being followed intensified a hundredfold with each step and I felt the presence of someone or *something* right behind me, following me down the stairs. Something malicious. I sped up and fumbled with the lock at the bottom door, all thumbs and no fingers. When I finally manged to open it, I launched myself into the falling snow and slammed the door shut behind me. Am I going mad? I wondered, as I walked the short distance back home, my footsteps muffled in the undriven snow. Is Parky now playing with my mind? Hallucinations for people who have Parkinson's is quite normal. I went through a stage of seeing black cats everywhere. This, though, was different, as I hadn't actually seen anyone, but just felt an overwhelmingly unpleasant presence next to me.

The next day I attempted to explain what had happened – or tried to – to the landlord.

'Paul, I was working late last night and …'

He looked at me quizzically and then smiled, 'So you met him?'

'*Him*?'

'Yes, the resident ghost.'

'So there *is* something here,' I said.

'Did he follow you?'

'He did. All the way down the stairs.'

'Anything else?' he asked.

I was still reeling with the fact that he, too, knew all about it. 'No,' I said.

'Well, in that case you're lucky.'

'Lucky how?'

The estate agent looked at me squarely, 'He grabbed me by my neck.'

I made a mental note to ask my neurologist if illusionary hauntings were also a symptom of Parkinson's disease. And another to find a different office.

Nothing could appease my anger at being powerless to help my beautiful girl. When you don't have a God to curse – as I did not – you're not sure where to aim your ire. Not that I started drinking too much, paid for sex with prostitutes, started gambling online or taking drugs, all of which regularly happen with sufferers of PD. I resented and blamed myself that this was happening to us all, while I seemed to be standing on the side-lines spectating. I would constantly joke and say things like, 'The reason I haven't started drinking too much is that I can't afford to. The same goes for drugs.' Truth be told, going off the rails was the furthest thing from my mind. I had no intention of crashing and burning in front of my children, nor did Ali deserve it. But Parky had other things planned for me.

With her Smurf's nose, blue eyes and full lips, Aggs looked just like me when I was about her age. When she was angry or about to cry, her bottom lip puckered out, as mine had as a little boy. I once showed her a faded picture of myself and asked her who it was, to which she pointed at herself and said, 'Me'. One of the worst things about my illness was not being able to give Aggie all the time and support that I could have, had I been well and able. Financially speaking, freelancers live by the seat of their pants as a matter of habit; sadly, I had never been the best forward planner and had not been shrewd enough to take out a life insurance policy – so I couldn't stop working when my diagnosis arrived. There are certain things in life you cannot be cavalier about. Health insurance is one of them. If you're reading this, are healthy and you have kids and no health insurance, then do yourself a favour, get on the internet today and for the price of a pint or two, you can rest assured knowing your monthly policy will cover you if you fall ill so you don't have to work and can address your condition head-on.

Ali took Aggs to most of her appointments with physios, speech therapists, mobility consultants, gait experts – the list was endless – while I kept grafting away to pay our huge mortgage. And when I wasn't researching travel guidebooks for Lonely Planet or on assignment for a newspaper – which was about a third of the year – I was back home writing up these books, updating the information on maps and refreshing the information about the safety of the particular country. It was all very intensive. I was also involved in corporate training in London, the US and the Middle East. Most of these training gigs required that I be in London for 9 a.m. start and to meet this requirement meant catching a 5 a.m. bus from Cirencester to London

Victoria. That was okay for the first two years of having PD, but then it began to take its toll, visiting me with the worst fatigue, where ordinarily I would have been fine. The work itself was fairly straightforward; it was just the journey time that was the problem.

Latterly, when my illness prevented me from doing Lonely Planet work, I found new and immensely satisfying writing work helping elite sportsmen and ex-Special Forces operators tell their stories in print as the co-author of their books. I've always been more interested in other people's stories than my own, so I was in my element.

The established advice for people with Parkinson's is, when you're tired go with it, don't try and fight it, just lie down and close your eyes for a bit. The problem is that when you're working directly with others and are suddenly feeling overcome by fatigue, you might be in the middle of a sentence, on your feet explaining something to a room full of people. You can't just sleep when you are busy working, and you have to fight every fibre in your body which is pleading with you to sleep on the nearest table.

Chapter 2

Finding My Inner Viking

For my Christmas present, my sister-in-law kindly bought me an Ancestry.com test which required me to spit into a test tube, then send it off to some laboratory so my DNA could be studied. The results would give me an idea where my ancestors originally came from. It sat on my shelf an awfully long time, but one day I finally got around to it, delivered the requisite spittle into a sealable plastic cup, placed it in the prepaid envelope and sent it off. It turned out that most of my ancestors were Vikings from Norway or Iceland, which pleased me no end; I've always had wings on my heels itching for adventure, and these brave people seemed to have the same problem, a need to explore. *Berserking* and pillaging, you'll be glad to hear, come way down on my list.

The other notable location revealed by my genetic foot-print was the Scottish Western Isles where the Norsemen had settled and become farmers; the main glut of them on the Isle of Harris where, curiously, Jim Morrison, the Doors singer's family hailed from (the clan of the McMorrisons!) and disappointingly orange Donny (Mr Trump). But there was another island with my ancestors' genetic stamp; its neighbour, Skye. I decided to read up on the Vikings in a little more depth.

What is it about those extraordinary Norsemen which lights the imagination like a flaming torch? To me, medieval times are bit dreary until from the fog of the late eighth century emerge the dragon-headed prow of the Vikings, heralding a period which was to last until the late eleventh century. The word *Norseman* (literally, man from the north) conjures up images of warriors with braided blonde hair framing fearless faces carved from granite, hoving to in longships with striped sails. The Vikings hailed from a brutally cold land bathed in the magic light of the Aurora Borealis. They brought danger, brutish charm and strange mystic rituals including sacrifices to the gods and ceremonial piss-ups quaffing tankards of mead to aid with storytelling. *Seior* was the practice of foretelling the future. They raped and pillaged, and fought with a level of ferocity it's hard to comprehend, believing that they were bound for the halls of Valhalla (a ramparted heaven for warriors killed in battle). Yet there were contradictions about these forbidding giants that are hard to square; yes, they were raiders, pirates and murderers, but they were also traders, explorers, storytellers, silversmiths, farmers and colonisers.

After they conquered and settled in the western isles of Scotland and elsewhere, they no longer needed to kill and raid; instead they became peaceful farmers of the land (much as they had been at home in Scandinavia before the raids began). Viking women were celebrated for their courage and ferocity, owned their own property and had the right to divorce their husbands, something unheard of in Europe at the time. The Norse people were also very hygienic, bathing at least once a week (!), brushing their teeth and regularly washing and combing those golden Scandi locks. When they weren't fighting, the Vikings were farming or fishing, and when they weren't doing either of these, they designed incredibly intricate silver filigree jewellery. They navigated by the stars and regarded the sea with the deepest reverence. They built hardy craft that would take them all the way across the Atlantic to discover America five hundred years before Columbus. They took enormous risks and regarded life as an adventure to be squeezed till the last drop came out. They ate a healthy diet with plenty of fish and fruit and veg, and kept themselves fit with daily exercise. But the one magic ingredient which allowed them to cover great distances by sea, and replenish their bodies with nutrition during these epic voyages, was stockfish: cod dried on racks in the sun and wind. Naturally salted by the sea air, it could last for five to seven years.

For centuries, Scandinavians from Iceland to Norway have been immersing themselves in ice pools for the purpose of bringing good health. Their ancient forebears, the Vikings, had a ritual to harden themselves and focus the mind called 'the ice hole'. They would lower themselves into a hole cut out of thick ice in the lakes and rivers beside which they lived. They taught themselves to sit calmly as their bodies became accustomed to the freezing temperature, knowing that the benefits far outweighed the discomfiture. It not only toughened them up, but by acclimatising themselves to the extreme cold it enabled them to sail vast distances where others would have lost their bottle.

One day soon, I wanted to go to Skye to wild swim and find my inner Viking! But I would need a proper angle to make it float with a broadsheet editor. I had to try and think of something.

It was now 2015. Nothing shifted my black mood and lifted my soul more dramatically than cold water swimming in a nearby lake, which was also used for sailing and triathletes (but only one or the other at any one time). I felt the benefits during and straight after each swim, every pore on my body tingling joyfully. I could feel the blood rushing around my shivering limbs, and my head pulsing. But most of all, I loved the calmness it brought out in me; for the first time in over three years of darkness I noticed that after each swim I experienced a brief window of serenity, where I was able to see the world free of anxiety through a more optimistic pair of eyes. It was like meditation without the required concentration. All this from swimming in a cold lake! It seemed a very small price to pay for achieving such vital equilibrium.

I used to feel similar after sparring in the ring, ridding my body of unnecessary stress and ill thought. Afterwards, it seemed as if my body was earthed but my spirit was light and free. The fear, if I had any, was gone. Ali used to say I looked as calm as a Zen monk after sparring. But wild swimming was even more powerful.

Along with a new friend of mine called Hugh, I started swimming three times a week, leaving a warm bed to shiver me timbers in a lake inhabited by moorhens and dark-blue fish. It was summer, and well worth the early start. Sleepy-eyed, we would regard the lake's mill-pond stillness, often topped in a fine mist, then lose our breath as we slid into its icy cool embrace. The initial panic soon cleared, but I found that diving straight in set my heartbeat racing a little too quickly; it was better to immerse yourself inch by inch and work your way gradually to full immersion.

I'm not terribly good at making new friends. I have a clutch of very old ones whom I have known for three decades, a couple of others from my acting days and a handful of fine people I've met across the world and with whom I've remained friends. Hugh, though, was just one of those people that you seem to click with effortlessly. We couldn't have been more different: as well as being a beekeeper he ran an investment company worth hundreds of millions. His brain worked in a very different way than mine, and yet we had a great mutual respect for each other.

It was so much nicer swimming in a natural body of water than doing laps in a chlorinated pool like a metronomic goldfish. Lake 32, whose perimeter was about a kilometre, was brilliant green in colour and so clear you could see fish flash like quicksilver beneath you as you swam from one fluorescent buoy to the next. Swimmers would glide past us in their wetsuits. Unlike the triathlon mob we never swam in wetsuits, preferring to wear just trunks. Partly because it robbed us of the benefits of cold water and partly because we were purists and you just didn't get a realistic drag whilst wearing a wetsuit, since the buoyancy in the neoprene pushes your legs up so you're more level in the water. While this is great for speed, you don't feel like you have as much of a workout as when you just go in in your trunks.

After the swim, with muscles aching, skin tingling and both with beaming smiles, we would tuck into a thermos of tea Hugh had thoughtfully prepared that morning, whilst sitting on the trunk of a downed tree that quickly became known as 'the philosophy log'. It was here that we would put the world to rights, talk about climate change, articles we had read in *Wired*, as well as swapping travelling stories. Occasionally we'd talk about Stoicism, an ancient school of thought I was increasingly relying on to help manage my negative thinking.

The four principles of Stoicism are justice, courage, wisdom and temperance. I desperately needed the courage to share my Parkinson's diagnosis with a friend and get it off my chest. But how do you tell someone something which will instantly disappoint them and reframe what they think of you? This was how irrational my thinking was back then. I seemed unable to reach out to others for help, either because I was too proud to admit my body had given in to this older person's disease (likely), or I didn't want to burden them (also likely). One of the hardest aspects of the confession was accepting that I was no longer physically the man I had been before. I was fast becoming a husk of a thing.

In 2013, we had shared our news of Agatha's condition with a choice number of our closest friends and family, and not wanting to bombard them with too much tragedy all at once, we kept quiet about my disease. I think it's fair to say we were a little embarrassed to admit that life seemed to have written a hex on our door. We disliked pity almost as much as the diseases we were having to accept as part of our life, and pity was exactly what we were likely to get were we to come clean about all our problems. I have a couple of friends who know me so well I think I could trust them with anything; in fact I know I can. The problem is the first person that I told about my diagnosis burst into tears and kept shaking his head, saying 'This is terrible, you of all people Rich. You're our rock … if it can happen to you. it can happen to any of us.'

I almost felt I should apologise. There is no doubt that those tears were made of pure compassion, but there was also an element of loss there too, not for me but squarely for him. I had been the reluctantly sporty one at school, the one who stepped in front of the rest of my pack when someone held a smashed bottle to block our way through an alleyway. I was supposed to be the fearless one, and now I was diminished, irrevocably on a downward slope.

The main principle of Stoicism is that you need only to focus on the things you have control of and you shouldn't waste your time worrying about something over which you've got no agency, like the economy or global warming, or developing cancer, or other's opinions of you, as there's nothing that you can do to change any of these. The only things that lie within your power to control are your opinions and the way in which you respond to any given situation.

In Stoicism we can choose to be brave, practise wisdom and do what is right. That's all very well, but I was having a problem squaring away my care and concern for my daughter, given that I had no control over it. How does any parent stop feeling bad about one of their children being ill just because there's nothing that they can do? I'm not picking a fight with Stoicism, because it helped me enormously, but there are limits to everything, and fine lines, caveats and grey areas.

I suppose Stoicism was saying, 'Look, if you can't change it, then at least just try and maximise it. Make the most of Aggs and your own time if you don't know how long either of you have got.'

One day, after my morning swim with Hugh, I was sitting at the desk in my office at the top of our house when I happened upon an internet page showing a woman swimming underwater in a rockpool of turquoise water. It was at a place called the Fairy Pools on the Isle of Skye, and she was being described as a wild swimmer. It was all pleasantly whimsical. I thought back to my DNA report and my Viking genes. Something was cooking in my brain.

That afternoon, I sat down and wrote a proposal for a trip to Skye, focusing on wild swimming, then sent it to some travel editors. I didn't mention my Parkinson's to the newspapers. I don't know why, as it would have been much easier to pitch. Maybe I was still carrying a level of shame. Outside, a brilliant spring sky radiated optimism and I thanked the universe that I still had interesting work.

My energy levels were being daily eroded by Parky. The disease's noticeable tremor was progressing up my right arm and now down my right leg. In my applied practice of being grateful, I reminded myself to be glad of the warm weather and the fact it was a writing day and so I didn't have to go to London on the 5 a.m. bus for training work. I thanked the universe, too, that the disease had not yet spread to my left-hand side, which it would inevitably do. I had even got into the habit of thanking the meds (all twenty of them and which I hated taking), as I gulped them down first thing in the morning. These turned my pee the colour of Lucozade and made it stink sharply of chemicals, but it seemed a small price to pay for a few hours of stillness. If I visited the men's room, I had to pee in a cubicle, otherwise to those relieving themselves next to me at the urinal, it looked like I was pissing kryptonite. The pills worked on and off, so I'd have a few hours in which I could almost rely on them to keep me still, but they could suddenly wear off without warning, leaving me unable to control the shakes. When I didn't have the shakes, I most definitely had dyskinesia, which causes my body to do the strangest things; like when reaching into a drawer to get some cutlery, one of my legs would shoot out behind me as if I was doing a Fred Astaire-like dancing move.

It was a game of positive thinking. I tricked my mind into thinking everything was okay, and that with the right attitude I could get through this. Some days, I was winning. Thinking that my time with Aggs was limited actually gave me a sense of appreciation. It wasn't that I started questioning the point of life, more that I began to see its evanescent beauty and realise its brevity. Life can disappear from under our feet at such short notice, and the more aware we are of this, the easier it is to try and look for the bonuses.

At each annual visit to the neurology wing in London's Queen's Square, I told my neurologist, 'I can't let this thing beat me. I'll try anything – I'll be a guinea pig on a drug trial, whatever.' The problem was that in order for my meds to mask the symptoms effectively, the volume

I needed to take was growing substantially. In line with the expected worsening of the condition over the coming years, I was also terrified of losing freelance work, be it as a travel author or as a corporate trainer. As time passed, the drugs were starting to lose their efficacy. If I had to stand up and address an audience – often in America, and with anything from fifty to one thousand people – I would be a bag of nerves. And when I was nervous, the tremor got worse, so it became a vicious cycle. As if it knew when I was about to go on stage, Parky would reliably take a hold of the right-hand side of my body, simultaneously vibrating my arm and leg. In my determination to hide the shaking for fear I would be labelled an embarrassment, I was giving Parky too much focus and empowering it. Just thinking about it caused my hand to shake as if I was holding a high-powered electric drill.

For one particular training company, I worked all over the world. The very first job I did for them was in Dubai back in 2013. It was here one of my work colleagues noticed I was dragging my right foot and that my right arm didn't swing when I walked. He pointed it out to me, suggesting I might want to get it checked out by a doctor. He said he had a friend who had Parkinson's with similar symptoms. I thanked him and told him I'd look into it.

It was now summer 2015 and I'd had the illness for four years. As ever, my chief concern was, 'How long have I got before I have to give up work and how will I feed my kids?' There was a popular saying I often used,

'Where attention goes, energy flows'. I was clearly feeding the disease with my thinking and limited energy, and the disease was most definitely winning.

I stopped looking at the lady 'wild swimming' in turquoise water as I heard something bumping up the stairs. That something stopped before the final top three where the stairs curled around a corner. My daughter burst into a fit of giggles: Agatha was the worst at keeping quiet.

'Is anyone there?' I asked and her blonde head popped up over the stairs like a jack-in-the-box, her brilliant blue eyes full of mischief, her smile revealing the gaps in her milk teeth. I loved these visits from her; it was a steep haul to the top of house for Aggs, given that her energy was zapped by her condition and her balance problems meant she was now falling more. I tried to stay in the present and not to think about the indisputable fact that we were both getting worse.

On 26 June 2016, Aggie's illness was finally diagnosed. She had developed 'Tubb4a H-abc'. The only doctor in the UK who knew what that was, Dr Livingstone, was based in Leeds where he had started a protein clinic for 'white matters' on the brain. Meeting him made some sense out of the chaos. So far, we'd been passed from pillar to post, and as Aggie's illness never halted for a second, we could never catch our breath.

Ali or I would often take Aggie out of normal school when the other kids were doing sports, so she could go horse-riding in Cheltenham, and she loved it. There was a helper on each side to catch her in case she lost balance and fell, and it was great for strengthening her core and a balm for her spirit and confidence. Aggie loves animals, and animals most definitely love her. If a friend came around with a dog, it naturally found its way to her and would sit by her side or lick her face. Animals have this lovely way of knowing if there's something wrong with you. Our cat Bessie would often come and lie on my shaking hand.

Aggie wore leg splints to help keep her feet from hyper-extending. We tried her on six different meds to stop her hands shaking, but even the tiny doses made her sick. 2016 was also the year when Aggie's stairlift was installed at our house. It represented a reality check for all of us that her disease was going to get worse and we were increasingly going to need the help of machines to move her around the house; and the house, though lovely, was not an open-plan modern layout that would have made things considerably easier.

In 2018, we took Aggie to a neurological diseases conference at McGill Hospital in Montreal. Whilst there she became part of a study run by the Boston Children's Hospital. Aggie did lots of tests, some of which measured her cognitive ability. It turned out she was super smart, off the scale. It was great to hear what we already knew, that she was sharp as a razor, but equally it made me so sad that my little girl had so much potential locked up inside her, yet was unable to find an outlet to express itself.

A section of the conference was about finding new ways to treat Tubb4a H-abc, and for the first time we heard about stem-cell therapy, and how it was fast becoming the new frontier of medicine. Stem cells are extraordinary: they can repair damaged brain cells and propel them into reactivity. We also got to meet other parents of kids with H-abc. Some of the children were older than Aggie, who at this point was ten years old. It's amazing what a little bit of hope can do; it can turn a desperate situation into one where there is a chance, however small, that something good might happen and progress might be made. This is what the promise of stem-cell research did for us. At its best it might transform Aggie's mind, and rebuild her natural abilities to walk and talk again.

Before we came to Montreal, I had been contacted by Darren Hardy, an ex-soldier who suffered from PTSD. He was originally from Belfast and had grown up through 'the Troubles' as a boy, when he witnessed knee-capping. His PTSD stemmed from his time in Iraq as a soldier. He was softly spoken and asked if he could come and meet me with regard to my writing a book with him. Apparently, he and his wife had found me online and read one of Tyson Fury's books which I had written with him. Darren said he really wanted to raise money for Aggie and also awareness about her largely unknown disease. About the same time, Ali met and began a dialogue with two mothers, Michelle and Amy, whose children also had Aggie's condition. They would talk for hours on end, cathartically sharing their stories with one another. In fact, they got on so well that they registered and started up a charity called 'The H-abc Foundation' with a GoFundMe page. It was the first time we had put our head above the parapet and talked to strangers about the nightmare of H-abc. Aggie got her own GoFundMe page.

Darren was a friendly guy with an honest, open face. He proposed to run five marathons back-to-back along the coast road in Dorset. Looking back and joining the dots together, his arrival into our lives was well timed. With a date set for the marathon run, we were asked to appear on Sky TV national news at about eight in the morning. It was surreal, trying to explain the complex areas of Aggie's brain which were affected by the disease, while millions of people were watching over their breakfast. This was alien territory for us but keeping quiet wasn't helping Aggs, so we had to grab every opportunity no matter how uncomfortable it made us feel. Another TV slot on the BBC arranged by an old friend who worked in PR involved the three mums of the charity meeting for the first time in Michelle's back garden. By then, the pandemic had appeared on the horizon and we all had to socially distance.

The other really significant development which gave us cause to hope was the creation of a biotech company, which was set up purely to find a cure for H-abc. It would take years to come to fruition, but if Aggs could hold on, it was possible they might find a cure or at least a medical intervention through gene therapy that would stop the disease in its tracks and go some way to restore the damage the disease had caused in her brain.

The mind is our own worst enemy in the way it insists on making comparisons with the past and obsessing over what might be in the future. In our case, with two degenerative diseases working 24/7, it was difficult not to fret about the future. I often reflected that before Aggie's and my diagnoses, I had so little to worry about; if only I had known the proportions of what was coming, I might have lived those moments more joyously. But what was the sense in looking back and thinking like that? It just made me feel worse.

Back to Skye and the Vikings. Despite being thrown in the deep end of a swimming pool at the age of five and told to 'swim!', I have always been a lover of water (not a bad thing, given my surname). Despite having the greatest respect for it, I've almost perished in its embrace on many occasions: like the time before I could swim when I sank to the bottom of a hotel pool having cried wolf that I was drowning one too many times to my exasperated parents (I was rescued by a vigilant Frenchman); or snorkelling in Mexico, when having spotted a shaft of sunlight at the end of a long underwater tunnel, I figured it to be a breathing hole, struck out for it and reached it, only to find there was no headspace to breathe and I had to fight my way blindly back as my vision clouded red like the closing curtains in a cinema before the film begins.

On another occasion, I was training solo in prep for the Brighton Pier-to-Pier challenge. I'd swum to a distant yellow buoy a kilometre out to sea in the English Channel when I was enveloped in thick fog and couldn't find my way back to the shore; with hypothermia closing in, I lost articulate control of my arms and legs. The long and short of all this was, if I was going to Skye to try and improve my Parky symptoms in mountain lakes and streams, I probably needed someone who could help me keep out of trouble.

Within a few days I had a pair of commissions for the Skye wild swimming story; one an *i news* feature and the other a six-page spread at *Coast* magazine. I then contacted the Scottish Tourist Board to see if they could give me any assistance on the trip, such as organising a hire car.

Summer, the lady at the Scottish Tourist Board, told me, 'Skye has more waterfalls, pools and elusive mountain tarns than a wild swimmer can dream of, but unless you know where to find these spots most of them will remain hidden. Fortunately, for you there's an expert guide called Matt Rhodes who lives on the island and knows it like the back of his hand. He'll maybe take you. Here's the number.'

I thanked her, hung up and called Matt, leaving a voice message. He called me back almost immediately.

'I'd be happy to take you on a one-day tour, Richard,' he said in a thick Lancashire accent.

'That's great news. By the way Matt, I've got early onset Parkinson's Disease, is that a problem?'

'Not for me it's not. I've taken blind people and people in wheelchairs into the water, so don't worry.'

'Do I need to bring any special kit?' I asked.

'Just bring yourself.' We arranged to meet me in four weeks' time in a car park beside the sea in Portree, Skye's capital. I was excited!

The next thing I did was to consult Google maps. It was about two-and-a half hours' drive from Inverness airport, where I'd pick up my hire car, to Portree, which was roughly speaking the girdle, or waist, of the island of Skye. The tourist board had kindly placed me in a bolthole called the Uig Hotel, which was a further half hour's drive north.

Skye's shape reminded me of a ragged owl with an enormous wingspan, colliding with the west coast of the mainland. The island, which belongs to an archipelago known as the Inner Hebrides, is connected to Scotland's north-west coast by a bridge and measures some 50 miles long and 25 miles wide. It is also the second largest island in Scotland after Lewis and Harris. No sooner had I crossed it than I felt a little different. How? I'm not completely sure and I may be making it up. Let's just say I felt lighter.

It was night time as I arrived in Uig, which sat on a small incline that gave a commanding view of the distant harbour of Uig, and a huddle of houses looking seaward across the bay, few of them climbing up the sharp hill behind. I should have felt exhausted by now; instead I felt slightly revived. And that was a good job, as I'd need every ounce of energy for what the next day had in store for me.

Chapter 3

The Climb to Coire Lagan

How to Win an Argument With Yourself

I wasn't sure how much walking would be involved that day, so I picked up a bottle of Lucozade and some Dextrasol energy sweets in Portree. With its handsome little square and pretty confection of pastel-coloured houses huddled around a small harbour on one side, and the picturesque bay on the other, it was delightful. From somewhere not far away came the plaintive shrill of bagpipes. I walked the short distance from the square to the car park and looked around for my wild swimming guide; it didn't take very long to pick him out among the tourists.

With his plaited beard, long hair roped in dread-locks and huge arms tattooed with wolves and skulls, Matt looked more like a Viking than a wild swimming instructor. But as we've seen, given that the island was settled by Vikings in the late eighth century – 'Skye' after all is derived from the Old Norse word for 'cloud' – his appearance seemed oddly appropriate. Matt wasn't a tall person, but he had the solidity of a rock: huge shoulders, and possessed of a quiet self-assured presence that made him seem bigger. His eyes were angular slits and as he smiled and held out a hand to shake mine, the morning sunshine caught his face and revealed one dark brown eye and one that was steely blue. As I would soon discover, he was considered by some locals to be even more *local* than them, such was his closeness to the land and waters of Skye.

Matt's car boot was spilling out with unruly neoprene wetsuit boots, dryrobes, chocolate bars, towels and rucksacks.

'Make yourself comfy, Rich,' he said and motioned me to climb into the car.

'We're going to head down to the south of the island first,' he said.

The landscape rolled by kaleidoscopically, changing from forest to moor, fen to hillock and meadow to mountain; it was as if Skye was many places rolled into one mass. One moment it was Mordor, the next Narnia, and by the time we reached the sickle sharp, saw-toothed range of the Cuillin mountains, the sun had come out and been eclipsed by raincloud at least twice in the space of an hour. It was as if Skye's epidermis was seal-hide rather than soil, for it seemed to shake off any evidence of a downfall within minutes. We parked up by a shoreline of black sand and Matt pointed up at the nearby hill segueing into mountain which in turn was summited by cloud.

There were wild flowers everywhere. 'Coire Lagan means the mountain lake, it's way up there.'

My neck cricked as I craned to take it all in. *Parky will never let me get up there,* I thought to myself. *I'll be dead on my feet!*

Matt's take on breathing when entering icy water was simple but effective, and unlike the technique advocated by Wim Hof, the Dutch 'Iceman', which prepares you for the cold by holding your breath for a long time at the end of a series of rapid breathings in and out, the Viking's advice was straightforward: 'Remember with your breathing, it's good to chat as you're going in to the water because your body will automatically control your breathing. You don't need to do long or short breaths … just keep talking, let your body do its thing.' We travelled light, each of us carrying a bag containing a dryrobe to change into to maintain our core temperature when we came out of the freezing water. This, plus a bottle of water and some energy bars. As we began our tramp up the mountain, I thought about Joe Simpson, the mountaineer who fell into a crevasse in the Andes in Peru after his fellow climber had (understandably) cut the rope he was suspended from in order to save his own life. Simpson, in agonising pain from a badly broken leg, had climbed out of an ice cave using his three sound limbs, and shuffled on his arse across miles upon miles of glacier. He had broken the enormity of his journey down into a series of smaller targets, identifying the next spot he would reach every 20 minutes.

Mindful of this, from here on I tried not to look up at the cloudy summit that seemed never to get any closer, but instead focused on nearby waypoints of granite, or cairns in the distance, then set off, keeping my eyes on where I was placing my feet. I think climbing a mountain is a fine metaphor for how we approach life. When you look up at the summit, it's disheartening to see how far you have to go. If you ponder the distance between yourself and your end-point, you immediately feel tired and defeated. But if you focus more on where you are now, putting one foot in front of the other, your mind will not be disheartened. Keep it local, keep your radius of attention small. Rome wasn't built in a day, but block by block, just as a mountain is scaled by putting one foot in front of the other. Our life needs goals – without them we have no purpose – and yes, my purpose was to reach the pool near the top of this particular mountain. In the meantime, though, there was the journey itself to focus on, waypoints to reach, the immediate landscape around us to soak up.

The brook babbling beside me and the crunching footfalls of my boots on the wet shale and slippery rock became my present soundtrack. I forgot about thinking how tired I was and focused instead on how lovely it would be to cool off eventually in the lake. What's that saying, 'Where attention goes, energy flows'?

Matt and I found ourselves chatting about cults and he disclosed to me that he and his wife had been brought up as Jehovah's Witnesses. They had met when they were

THE CLIMB TO COIRE LAGAN

fifteen, having both grown up under the controlling faith, then had plotted their escape and left together. He referred to it as 'the religion'.

We must have been climbing for an hour-and-a-half, maybe two, by the time we'd *almost* reached Coire Lagan, a mountain loch fortressed by pinnacles of rock. I looked back down the way we had come; far below I could see the black sand beach at Glenbrittle from where we started our walk, and had then progressed through boulder meadows, bracken and purple heather, the air tinged with the fecund smell of wild garlic and thyme. Matt pointed to a distant channel in the black bay from where 1,200 years ago, the Norsemen had dragged their nimble boats on to land. They had flat hulls which enabled them to sail up rivers in water just a few feet deep.

By this time, I had refilled my water bottle for the umpteenth time in the mountain spring, and my legs were so tired with incessant climbing they were now wobbling, reminding me of when I used to box and had nothing left in the can come the end of a round. My legs had never been my strongest asset, even as a rugby player and 400-metre runner. I was definitely an arms man. Breathless, I asked Matt, 'How far is it to the top?'

'One more push will see us there,' grinned Matt, before disappearing into a fog bank that was moving ominously towards us. A few minutes later, I was on all fours crawling over Velcro-textured gabbro rocks, the wind howling like a banshee. I couldn't see beyond the end of my fingers, but rather than panic I decided to sit down and wait until the fog had rolled on. You can begin to panic very quickly when you're up a mountain and cannot see a thing, I reminded myself that the mist wouldn't last forever, I was sufficiently warm and that I had water; all of which would allow me to sit out the weather front until it had moved on. I also had a guide who was just on the other side of that fog. Being caught in a weather situation is a lot like life itself; when things get tough we are inclined to panic and make poor decisions based around getting somewhere – anywhere else than here – when all we really need to do is trust that the eye of the storm will move on. We just need to sit with where we are and plant ourselves firmly on the ground.

Shortly, the white wall of fog shifted and I saw that Matt was only about 20 yards ahead and we were near the top of the rise. He watched me closely to double-check I had enough puff to get me up the last bit and then, after another five minutes' climb, I was able to glimpse Coire Lagan for the first time – or part of it – because the rest of the loch was completely obscured in mist, the water opaque and forbidding, with unearthly yellow weeds beneath the surface. The lake on a good day is the colour of blue coral, but right now it wasn't exactly screaming, 'Welcome!' Rather, it looked like the kind of place you might interrupt a couple of witches mid-ritual, or witness a sword rise up from the water's surface.

'The harder it is to reach, the wilder the swimming,' declared Matt. At an altitude of 1,930 feet, I hoped this

qualified. A seasoned ice swimmer and long-time resident of Skye, nothing seemed to worry him, and this quiet
confidence in turn became infectious.

I would learn a lot from Matt. There were of course the
basics regarding kit – never forget the dry changing robe,
the towel, neoprene booties and hat to keep your extremities from losing heat and, easy for beginners to forget,
plenty of layers for *after* swim, not to mention a whistle to
attract attention if you get into trouble – not something
I had to worry about swimming with the Viking – and
a brightly coloured hat and tow flow to alert any passing speedboats to your presence. And last but not least, a
thermos with something warm in it for when you emerge
from the freezing water. Then, there were the techniques,
such as acclimatising *before* the swim by taking gradually
longer daily cold baths and showers, aiming to spend 30,
then 60 seconds immersed in them. He taught me to avoid
beginner's errors: taking your first wild swim in winter, or
jumping straight in, an action liable to cause cold water
shock, a condition which causes a rapid increase in heart
and blood pressure and can result in a cardiac arrest in less
than a minute. He taught me to spot the signs of incipient
hypothermia, the shaking, loss of motor control and disori-
entation that take a grip when the body's temperature falls
dangerously low. But for all that, Matt also taught me that
if the right precautions are taken and with the right mind-
set, it will all be worth it. The benefits – I hoped, and
medical institutions such as the Mayo Clinic suggested

– might include reduced inflammation and muscle soreness, an elevated mood as your body produces 'feel-good' endorphins, a heightened immune system, better mental and physical resilience and improved cognitive function. To maintain your core temperature in wild swimming, your heart also has to work harder to circulate blood around your body, which improves your cardiovascular fitness, as well as strengthening your immune system by producing more white cells which are what the body uses to fight off infection

The future benefits seemed largely hypothetical and the stretch of freezing cold lake very real. We stripped down to our trunks and stood at the edge of the black water as Matt explained the best way to handle icy water. 'Get used to the cold in three stages,' he said, as the wind whistled around us. 'First immerse yourself up to your knees, then to your waist, and then the rest of your body,' he instructed, his dreadlocks neatly folded into an oversized swimming cap that made him look like the lovechild of Beowulf and the creature from Alien.

I dallied by the pool's edge, its water sloe-black and those anaemic yellow reeds beneath its surface like grasping bony fingers wanting to pull me down.

'Come on,' said Matt breaking my thoughts, 'time to freeze your bollocks off.' Then it was dry-robe off and into icy water so cold it made my feet and fingertips burn. We moved slowly through the shallows and I fought my body's screaming urge to leap out and howl, my breath quickening with shock. This was my first taste of the cold water shock which often kills unprepared people jumping into cold water rivers and the sea. I counted to thirty, then stepped up to my waist as instructed. Shortly after, the mist opened to briefly reveal the remainder of the mountain rising above us towards an unseen summit.

I was up to my neck in the bleak waters of Coire Lagan and my body had started to adjust to the temperature, rapidly circulating blood to keep me alive. By the time I was out of the water, and into the dry-robe with a chocolate bar wedged in my mouth (for much needed sugar), I felt utterly fantastic, my skin vital and tingling, my heart pumping like a teenager's. It no longer mattered that the lake was so creepy and laced in thick mist, or that it had started to pour down. Inside, my soul felt it had had a spring-clean and the sun was shining again.

Who says you're finished? You've just walked/climbed for 2½ hours almost 2,000 feet up a mountain to swim in your first freezing loch … not bad for an old boy with Parkinson's.

For the first time since I couldn't remember when, I felt re-connected to my body again, and the feeling that once more anything was possible. The climb and swim up here had briefly blown away some of the cobwebs which had gathered these last few months through stress and anxiety worrying over Aggie's worsening state. Yes, I was powerless to control the speed at which scientists found a cure for either one of our illnesses, but I could at least try and make the most of the time we still had together. My existence felt more like a gift than a punishment. I remembered what the Stoic and Roman emperor, Marcus Aurelius said, 'Think of yourself as dead. You have lived your life. Now take what's left of it and live it properly.'

As we began our descent, I felt like a different person, lighter and clearer in myself. Strangely, I felt warm inside too, as if the cold water had given me a toasty aura. *But do I have to climb a mountain and freeze in a lake every time I want to feel this good?* I wondered. Whether it's a plunge or a long swim, so long as it is a natural place where you can immerse yourself in cold water and reap the après-dip benefits of your body releasing serotonin (the 'happy chemical' our brains produce), that's really all that matters.

'Wild swimming is not about who is the quickest and swims the furthest, at least not in my book,' said Matt. 'It's more the enjoyment of someone else's company and the conversation. Then there's the challenge of resisting the burning cold water, then sharing the euphoria afterwards. But it's the clarity that I get from it which is the best. Whatever inner turmoil I might be going through, this just seems to sort me out.'

'Another thing I love is winning an argument with myself,' he added. 'Before you get in, your mind has a conflict with you, telling you, "Not to get in, it's too cold, too overcast." But when you don't listen to it you get a sense of satisfaction when you do go in. Like you've won. It's a great feeling, winning the argument with yourself. Nobody can stop you.'

I warmed to Matt quickly: there was no superflu-
ous chatter to fill natural silences, and no bullshit about
him. As we followed the slippery track downwards past
rain-sodden sheep, passing other climbers making the
ascent, the afternoon sun a limpid yellow blanketed in
cloud, Matt pointed to a man-made channel far below in
the bay, 'That's where the Vikings used to land.'

I pictured them in their dragon-headed longships, mooring up after a treacherous crossing from Norway. Their flat
hulls allowed them to travel upstream in very shallow water,
which made them perfect for striking inland up rivers when
they were raiding. Their prow was the same as their stern,
allowing for a quick escape in reverse using oar power.

On average, the journey from Norway to here took
about a week. The Viking longships could travel quickly,
up to 740 nautical miles per day if the wind was in their
favour. But I wondered how they handled the longer
journeys, like the three-week sail to Greenland or to
modern-day America. Just how had they broken the journey up so it wasn't too intimidating? And how frightening
must it have been sailing into unknown uncharted seas
when there was no land to be seen for weeks on end? I
guess they just had to trust in their capabilities and their
gods to watch over them and grant them safe passage.

I said goodbye to Matt, feeling like I had made a new
friend. In my job as a travel writer I meet a lot of folk,
many of whom I intend to stay in touch with, but never
do. But I had a hunch Matt and I would meet again soon.

Chapter 4

Sea Cave of Flodigarry

Catastrophising

I needed a reason to return to Skye, but I couldn't just disappear off on a whim. I had responsibilities and it had to be worth it financially. Maybe I put it out to the universe to get me there – don't know – but whatever it was that gifted me the reason, just a few months later an opportunity came up. I was to write a self-help book with an ex-Special Forces operator who was appearing at the time opposite Ant Middleton on TV's 'SAS: Who Dares Wins'. They were filming on the island next to Skye, and on Skye itself.

We will talk about something I call 'joining up the dots', in Chapter 12. In essence, it means that there are certain events in your life which are predetermined and where one thing leads to another almost as if there is a magical unseen pathway. But because life is designed to be a mystery, we can't shine a light on the future dots and simply follow them. Instead, we have to trust that our life has meaning, that the events in it have a purpose and that we are going in the right direction. In order to help get this book written, a book I had no inkling of writing at the time, the universe had placed Matt in my path. Now it placed Ollie Ollerton. I liked Ollie from the word go. For my interview with him we sat in Soho House in London, surrounded by media types doing their best to look interesting. I was there to discuss ghost-writing his next book with him. Ollie looked like anybody else really; it was only when he popped to the loo that you could tell by his easy gait that he was fit for his years, and the way he walked on the balls of his feet betrayed his athleticism.

We cut to the chase quickly, discussing what the book would be about and how he wanted it presented. I was really impressed; his vision was very clear and I got this excited feeling in my gut that it was a book that I wanted to write. It wasn't going to be your average special forces book by any means. We shook hands, and I left him in the bar with his soft drink and the media gang. I didn't hear from Ollerton's publisher for a couple of weeks and I began to think that maybe he'd gone for another writer, as is sometimes the case.

To my genuine surprise, the first two books I had ghost-written had both become *Sunday Times* bestsellers. I have no idea how: I just did my best on them as I do with every book that I write. There really is no rhyme or reason as to what makes a bestseller and what keeps a perfectly brilliant book out of that much coveted Top

10 stable. Obviously, the currency of the author counts for a lot in non-fiction. For instance, Tyson's book had sold like hotcakes: he was the world champion for the second time, and was in between the second and third of his trio of fights with Deontay Wilder. You couldn't get any more current than that. And yet a book about the values inculcated by the Military Academy at Sandhurst, which I'd been asked to write eight months earlier, and which had seemed such a modest little tome, had done unexpectedly well – it made it to number seven in the *Sunday Times* bestseller list, despite not being obviously linked to a current news story or celebrity.

Against my usual judgment I called Ollie direct. He was very nice and a bit surprised to hear from me, 'Sorry you've not heard yet, Rich. I told the publisher I wanted you to write it the same afternoon we met. Let me make a call.'

He came back within five minutes.

Once a special forces operator, always a special forces operator, I thought as his number flashed up on my mobile.

'Rich, I've just called them. If I don't do the book with you, I said I'm not doing it.'

'What did they say?'

'They were meaning to make you an offer last week. It's just bureaucracy holding things up. So this is the gig,' he said, his voice shifting gear. 'If you can come out to the islands on the last weekend of October – oh, sorry, we are filming on the little island of Raasay but I'd like to get off it for the weekend – I can book us an Airbnb on Skye.'

'Skye?' I asked dumbfounded.

'Yes, do you know it, Outer Hebrides?'

'A little,' I said.

'Right, well if you can come out on that weekend, I will have just wrapped filming the regular series there, and we can work like nutters over the weekend before I return to the island to film *I'm a Celebrity ... Get Me Out of Here!*, I mean *SAS Who Dares Wins Celebrity*. Whatever it's bloody called!' He laughed.

I was over the moon, firstly because I liked Ollie; he'd been one of the quieter, least barky personalities among the ex-SAS staff on the show, and secondly, because he'd lived and survived a fascinating life, and he was very honest about his struggles with drink and depression. But mainly it was because I would be going to Skye in autumn, my favourite time of the year, and I could go wild swimming again on my favourite island.

We humans have been on this earth for 300,000 years, and just 15,000 years ago we were still being hunted by carnivores. On the timeline of evolution, that's a mere blink of the eye, so it's understandable we are still programmed to be on the look-out for something that's going to eat us. Because we are hardwired to expect danger, this makes us easily feel threatened and our jumpy thinking catastrophises, blowing many otherwise solvable problems out of proportion. For instance, I had begun the day feeling like shit, thinking that Ollie's book would not come through, neither would the other books that I was waiting to get greenlit by publishers. Left to my own devices, I catastrophised. But in this case I got so sick of doom-mongering, that I actually made myself snap out of listening to the negative voice I was beginning to believe, and made that call to Ollie. I was so glad that I had gone against the usual grain of just leaving it up to the whim of fate, the 'if it's going to happen it will happen' school of thought. The way I see it, 'if it isn't for you, it won't pass you.' Instead, I followed my gut instinct about Ollie: he was a good guy and we'd made a connection, so of course we were going to work together.

Just as we can use our imagination to visualise something good, when left 'untended' that same imagination will work against us. Often, when presented with an opportunity disguised as a challenge, we defer to the fear rather than going for it. However, this type of fear is more insidious: it's not an absolutely and immediate feeling, as in 'you've just been punched in the nose in a boxing ring' type of fear, no this is a different form of fear, low-level fear which might be disguising itself under the banner of common sense, ensuring that whatever the opportunity is, you say 'No!' to it. 'No, that's not for you, you're a little bit old to be doing that now,' or 'It's too good to be true, and besides, that will involve too much change to my life.'

Trust me. Your brain will make up myriad reasons why you shouldn't do something.

If only we can muster the courage to embrace these opportunities and go with them – even if they are taking us out of our comfort zones – they have the potential to point our lives in the direction that would make us the most happy. Eight months earlier, I had been asked to write a book on the values of the Royal Military College Sandhurst which were transferable to ordinary civilians. I met up with a pal whose son played rugby with mine. Many years earlier he had been to Sandhurst and was still a successful career soldier. He was very organised, as you'd expect, and was waiting for me with a pint and his own copy of a book on the academy, which is given to each cadet on their first day. 'Read this, it'll tell you all about the values.'

I was in a panic and working myself up to saying no to the challenge. 'I don't think I can write this, they need someone who's been a soldier,' I said uncertainly.

He looked at me square on, 'They need someone who can write. Listen, you've been given an opportunity, so grab it. I know you're going to write a brilliant book.'

Even though I had already signed a contract and agreed to hand the book in by a certain date, I had been talking myself out of it. I was prepared to stay in my comfort zone, one which wasn't actually that comfortable at all; it was tiring me out with too much travel for Lonely Planet, for not enough funds, and with too much training work in

London, which meant absurdly early starts to get there for the start of the day, which made my shakes obviously bad in public and in turn humiliated me. And then I felt like shit. This opportunity and newfound discipline of ghost-writing would allow me to work from home, and would pay me more to do so. Thankfully, it was much too late to back out on the Sandhurst book. To hell with comfort zones.

I don't think we are designed to be comfortable. Remaining in a predictable place ends with us dying choked by things that we don't need, and trying to plaster over the wound of inner emptiness with cars and possessions we think would make us happy and complete. The essence of courage and adventure is instead already within us, but something holds back many of us at from diving in. The term 'comfort zone' is a misnomer, it's less comfortable and more a place of dissatisfaction. Leaving such a place to push yourself into the unknown is the first step to waking up to yourself.

Wild swimming is the perfect expression of working through short-term discomfort for long-term gain, and by God it wakes you up! When you first slip into a freezing river or lake and feel immediately threatened by the bite of the cold water on your naked flesh, your mind screams 'Get out!', and 'This is unpredictable and dangerous for your health.' But if you trust the process and breathe through and beyond this hysterical voice, the fear quickly passes, and with it the pain of the cold. Soon enough, you realise that you're really not going to have a heart attack.

Then the fun starts, the water becomes your friend; your thinking is under control, your heart is pumping blood away from your extremities and your skin is tingling. Let's for the moment forget about all the science explaining what is happening in chemical and biological terms; I personally believe that on a spiritual level wild swimming reconnects us to our inner self, to the seat of the soul where we feel comfortable in our skin. It's only all the white noise and our own thinking that steals us away from the peace of our inner selves, and the fact that we have become used to the theft.

Our inner Viking looks at the watery horizon and yearns to know where it can lead him. Yes, we may still be programmed to look constantly over our shoulder, but the Vikings experienced fear and the same human misgivings about the unknown as we do. They just chose to push the boundaries and pass through their fear. Adventure is still very much in our nature; I would go so far as to say it's essential to our development. We need to follow its call to new experiences and then bask in their afterglow.

If we can embrace the unknown and keep moving through fear, we become stronger, fuller versions of ourselves, creating something new in the darkness and the unknown. To change anything in our lives we have to be prepared to step away from the predictable when the call comes. Because, like an exotic animal which briefly crosses your land, it might do so only once in a lifetime.

Most people on their deathbeds regret that they haven't taken a few more risks in their life. I look back and sometimes think I took too many risks. But there's a middle ground, a place of calculated risks, and well thought-through ventures to which I wish I had been more open when catering for things that could go wrong, like unseen illness. Who was I to think that I would get through life without a murmur? My son is thinking of becoming a free-lancer, and I believe he has the right mentality to thrive in that world of uncertainty, but there are things he can do to protect himself, like getting life cover before it's too late.

I'm uninsurable now.

Don't get me wrong. I have had, and still have, a rewarding writing career for which I'm very grateful, but I just wish I had looked ahead and planned a bit more. I think I was perhaps too trusting in my talents, and that life would deliver up something unexpectedly good at the last moment which would keep my family forever in clover. That is yet to happen. The thing with fantasy and reality is there's a disconnect that needs to be managed through hard facts if the two are to coalesce and become one. And you can only do that by being brutally honest with your-self, something I'm learning through illness.

Despite the fact I took as many career risks and personal risks, I wouldn't change any of it. That is who I am and I've been true to it, whether in boxing, travelling to dangerous places, or choosing infamously precarious careers like acting and writing. I just wish that I had cleared my desk of all the shit beforehand. By this I mean organised my finances, so I wasn't wasting valuable energy worrying. I went to college, did a degree in English and ended up becoming an actor. Not the best plan. Unless you know for sure the golden Lottery finger is shining directly on you, that's resting a lot on Chance's shoulders. If you are planning on doing something for the rest of your life or even for the next ten years, it's a major investment of time, so don't float passively on the ocean of hope – create your own current and take a hand in realising your own destiny.

If you were going to climb a mountain, you'd need to sit down and plan your route, and have a contingency route if that first one got blocked. You would have your kit, which would be vital to keep you warm and help you up the mountain; your carabiners, ropes, crampons, etc. And next, but not least, you'd have to pick your fellow climbers, but only those who you trusted with your life to help you if you got into trouble. In short, you'd have to be prepared. The life of an actor, writer or artist should be the same, with safeguards and alternative routes planned out. When so many of you are going for the same job, you have to learn to deal with failure and move on. And you have to learn to be true to yourself so you don't get swallowed up by whatever world you're in.

Once you have your shit together and know where you are financially, then you are in a healthy and freed-up space to say 'yes' to destiny's opportunities. I think the secret to reaping the most enjoyment from our days is to try and live with an element of risk and spontaneity, all of which wild swimming can deliver, as each new spot you visit is its own fresh adventure. And there is plenty that can go wrong, which adds some spice to it.

When your life feels dull, and every day a repeat of the one before it, you feel your soul dip with disappointment like a dog you promised a walk to but never got round to. The magic of wild swimming is that it costs nothing other than transport to get you there, and it requires no great mental effort; you just climb in your car, call a mate, get yourself into the water and then let nature do the rest.

Wild swimming in cold water causes the body to release endorphins, which are its natural mood boosters. I've been in the worst moods, ones that could have spiralled into depression had I not acted quickly and dragged myself into the nearest river, only to feel that remarkable sense of release and evaporation of negative thoughts. If you can form a habit of it, even better, as you not only get used to it to it physically and mentally, getting in no longer feels like a trial and it becomes second nature and a vital part of your day.

I called Matt almost as soon as I was off the phone from Ollie. I really hoped we could catch up on my next visit to Skye in the autumn. Matt answered immediately, and weirdly knew who I was before I even said it was me, 'Hello mate, how are you?'

'I'm good, thanks. How are you keeping?'

'All good. All good,' he answered.

After I explained to him what I was going to be doing on Skye, how long I'd be there and wondered if he'd be free to go for a swim Monday morning, we arranged to meet in the car park in Portree, just as we had last time.

Time can always be relied upon to gallop along, and before I knew it, it was time to go to Skye to meet Ollie Ollerton. It was autumn now, and the drive down from Inverness was through a pallet of gingernut and yellow-leaved trees and lochs that looked their glassy best beneath pearl blue skies. As it began to get dark, the hire car sped over 'Bifröst', the bridge that leads to the home of the gods in Viking lore. Actually, it was Skye Bridge, but the charge of energy I felt as I landed on Skye was palpable, and for some reason I always thought of the Vikings as soon as I got there.

It was Thursday evening by the time I met Ollie. I dumped my bags at the Airbnb and we repaired to a swish Indian restaurant to talk. The next day we were up fairly early, and we worked all day and late into the night. This was par for the course for the remainder of the weekend. Come Monday morning, Ollie slinked out ninja-quiet to catch the ferry to the tiny isle of Raasay, the only sign of his departure being the crunch of gravel beneath his black Land Rover's tyres. I hadn't so much as looked out the window at Skye for the last three days; we'd been that involved with his book I'd barely come up for air. But now I saw it all afresh, and looking very different than on my last visit.

Fired in autumn's forge, the island's former landscape of greens and purples had now been transformed into mellow coppers and golds. And the sea, retaining for a brief time the heat of the summer months, was also at its warmest – a tolerable though still feisty 12 degrees centigrade. In short, it was the perfect time for wild swimming and come 11 a.m. that morning, I was headed back in the water with the Viking of Skye.

As ever, we met in Portree car park. Matt was softly spoken and immediately easy company. He possesses a rare ability to pick the right body of water to suit the ability and fitness of his guest. And though he appeared relaxed at the prospect of my following him down a cliff face that day to reach the cave below, he watched me out of the corner of his eye with the keen care of an Anatolian Shepherd Dog checking its flock every few seconds.

But there was a problem, or at least one I kept confined in my head. I had a funny feeling in my gut that day and it was twisting around like a snake in a jar of butterflies; a kind of foreboding that something bad was going to happen. Clearly, my gut and brain were conspiring against me. Our destination that bright blue morning was the sea cave of Flodigarry. True, it was one of the more challenging wild swims on the island, but equally Matt knew that I was a strong swimmer and still liked to challenge myself. It was a calculated risk, but this is precisely the Viking's skill; he is able to assess your level of capability, and compare it to what you think your capability is; sometimes the two are not compatible! With this particular challenge, he was very clear in imparting the information I needed, to make it as safe as possible.

The place had an ancient presence. Apparently in pagan times sacrifices were performed at the sea caves. *Human sacrifice?* It preyed on my mind. I tried hard not to think of the Wicker Man and Edward Woodward's character burning inside a wooden effigy up on a hillside. Why was I so discombobulated and jumpy today?

'Something bad is going to happen to you or Matt,' said a voice in my head. 'One of you isn't coming out of that cave.'

I pressed pause on that suggestion and dialled back on the catastrophising.

Maybe because you've been working flat out for the last couple of days, and on all three nights you went to bed late and got up early, so you're a little burnt?

Finally, a voice of reason. The butterflies settled down a bit.

Shortly after, we crossed the last field before we came to an abrupt stop in front of a near-vertical cliff face covered in wet grass. Matt pointed down to Flodigarry cave. It was on a black boulder-strewn beach, its entrance shaped like a ziggurat dagger. Scattered around the cave's entrance, about were ropes of orange bull-kelp. Wave after menthol-green wave rushed into the cave's mouth, thundering in its echo chamber. The sea was trying to forbid us from entering the underworld.

I looked at the rocks far below. If I needed a good reason to be afraid, I now had one; one silly mistake in our descent and we could end up broken to pieces on them before we were even in the cave. We began to pick our way down the cliff, holding on to tussocks of grass to steady us. So long as I kept moving, vertigo, anxiety and fear were kept at bay. Busy people who are preoccupied doing something they enjoy, something that challenges them, are less likely to experience anxiety. A rolling stone gathers no moss.

At the base of the cliff, Matt looked for a break in the watery maelstrom, one sufficiently long enough for us to leap into the swell and swim quickly into the cave. My safety lay entirely in his hands – choose the wrong moment between sets and we'd both be dashed against the cliff.

Now I was poised and still, the fear had returned and wouldn't go away. It doesn't matter if you're a prince or a pauper, fear has the same effect on all of us. It seizes the gut and gives you this kind of jellified feeling in the abdomen. This is the lesser known sibling of fight and flight, and it's called freeze. I used to get it an awful lot when I first started boxing sparring. When faced with an unbeatable foe that you have no chance of winning, your body turns to literal mush, numb and unresponsive. Everything shuts down, while your brain is desperately figuring out what it's going to do.

Matt broke my thoughts, 'Ready, Rich? After the next wave, we're going in,' he said. 'Now remember, the incoming wave will try and suck you out to sea, so once you're in the cave grab hold of something.' I knew that if I failed to hold on and started disappearing out to sea, Matt would be there in a flash to join me. Even so, my mouth was dry and coppery as I watched his tattooed legs disappear into the drink. I had to follow. I took the plunge.

Having avoided being caught and dragged out in the current by holding on to a circular pillar of rock, I hauled myself up and sat Gollum-like on a ledge. Like a sci-fi movie set, the interior of Flodiggary cave was otherworldly, with cooled magma corridors and a ceiling of gothic pipe organs made of basalt. I was hypnotised by the roaring sea eternally filling up and ebbing from this ancient place, swirling and frothing in pink rock pools that it had fashioned over millennia. In this moment, in the church-high darkness, within this circular rhythm of nature, my mind had stopped thinking and my fear had gone away. Buoyed up by the minor triumph of not being carried out to the Orkneys, I felt somehow bigger.

Even Parky, the spiteful condition that stole my breath by night and humiliated me by day, had briefly gone, washed away by nature's cold-water therapy. As we caught a break between the hammering waves and escaped the surreal interior world of Flodiggary, I felt elated. I had summoned my inner Viking, passed through the negative thinking that had tried to talk me out of exploring the cave, and as a result I felt more like my real myself again.

Plato, the Athenian philosopher, believed that like a charioteer our mind is drawn by two horses: a positive one with a natural wisdom of where it needs to go; the other undisciplined and lazy, bent upon sabotaging the first horse. If we can learn to be aware of when the bad horse is biting, says Plato, we can reject the fear and anxiety it produces and let the good one take us to contented pastures. With practice comes wisdom and self-awareness. Once you get wise to spotting where the fear comes from, you can choose to sidestep it.

As we climbed back up the grassy cliff, I was thinking *When we look back on our lives, how much of it has been spent in a place of fear for things that never came to pass?*

Matt sparked up a rollie and offered me one. 'Right pal,' he said, 'we've got time for one more special pool before you head off the island of mist.'

Chapter 5

Rha Falls

Mid-Life Crisis

The sun came out as we headed north, biblical spears of light shooting down from the clouds and lighting on a huddle of deserted crofting houses. Shortly, we arrived at the stunning Lealt Falls, parked up and walked down a vertiginous cliff pathway with dizzying drops to the sea below. After a 20-minute descent, which was less than friendly to bad knee joints, we reached the bottom of the cliff at sea level, where the Lealt river empties its load into the Sound of Raasay. From here we followed the river upstream for about 10 minutes until we arrived at the magical falls. This was a peat river the colour of whisky. Sunlight danced over the frothing waters, bringing with it a chill from the sea. I felt very alive and fortunate to be here.

From the viewing point far above in the car park, tourists could see the top tier of the Cascades, the waterfall, but because of the rich vegetation around it they had no view of us whatsoever. Having an entire waterfall to yourself is a rare indulgence.

We walked a few miles north to Brother's Point, the most easterly point of the island. Basically a tussocky peninsula about the size of a football pitch, from it you can turn around and take in the utter drama that is northern Skye, the Old Man of Storr and the basalt cliffs forming the backdrop. At Kilt Rock, so called because the vertical formations of the basalt cliff look like the creases in a kilt, we parked up and had a coffee from a mobile café. From the top of the cliff there were splendid views of Raasay island opposite, and more immediately, down below huge boulders that over millennia had fallen in the sea, around them irises of turquoise. There was also a permanent sign showing a picture of the carnivorous 170 million-year-old dinosaur found preserved in these rocks.

Nearby, a lone bagpiper played. I don't remember the first time I ever heard bagpipes play, but I think it struck me as an unpleasant, wheezing scream. But now as I listened to it, it seemed to soothe me and touch my heart, as if it connected me to a deeper history of the island.

In the northerly village of Uig, Rha Falls is a magical and dramatic cascade surrounded by a thick wood of trees, and is best visited in sunshine which penetrates the over-head vegetation and dapples the water. The pool which sits beneath the waterfall is a good size for swimming; however, it's also incredibly murky because the water passes through peat which gives it a curiously reddish colour like a cup of Rooibos tea. I must admit peat is not my favourite kind of water to swim in when compared with say, aquamarine. There's another reason. Every time I am in the clutches of peat water, I am reminded of death. That sounds dramatic? I'm a wannabe free diver and love to get to the bottom, and yet when I put my head underwater in a peat river or lake, after a few feet the water goes from ruddy to absolute black, and it is like being suspended in a kind of purgatorial death, like 'the sunken place' in the film *Get Out*.

We all die a little bit, or at least shed a skin, when we reach middle age. To pass to the next physical stage of their life, one in which they no longer produce eggs, women must go through the menopause, a difficult time of hot flushes, night sweats (often during the day), mood changes, rage, bad sleep and difficulty concentrating (to name a few of the many symptoms). Meanwhile, middle-aged men wrestle with their own mid-life challenge. Namely, who the hell are they? Growing into our new skin and becoming an older man is a process that starts in our late forties and accelerates in our early fifties and presents a series of rapids that many guys struggle to navigate. Partly because the skin we have worn through our thirties and forties is now showing definite signs of wear and tear, many of us feel as if our best days are behind us. Maybe work has plateaued in terms of how far we can rise in our company, or perhaps the business of earning money has lost its glamour and we are feeling as if something is missing, despite the nice car, the lovely house which we worked so hard for, or maybe we have developed some horrible illness. Once the kids have found their teenage tribe, gone to college or started making their own families, we can find ourselves suddenly alone with just our wife or partner, our social circles smaller than they were ten years before. Women are much better at making new friends than men. Is it because they're better at being vulnerable than we are? I don't have the answer to that.

It can be a difficult time as far as vanity goes, too. By now most of us have lost a fair amount of hair, and our best-looking days are suddenly behind us. It's nature's little trick, because as fifty-somethings we are no longer required to re-populate the species. You only need to be good looking for a certain period of time, it seems. It can also be a period of spiritual bankruptcy, when members of our family begin to pass away, and we no longer know where we sit within the universe. And this is often topped off by a loss of purpose, in which we no longer have any meaningful goals to motivate us on a day-to-day basis.

More men commit suicide between the ages of forty-five and fifty-four than in any other age bracket. But why? I think it's down to many of us not feeling prepared or ready to accept these devastating effects of growing older. That and the lack of identity that often comes with ageing. Who and what am I now? It's as if we can't answer that. We're too old to be young and too young to be old!

Since that knee problem stopped us playing five-a-side once a week, or training for a triathlon, life has become a little bit too sedentary and the chances of fitting into those jeans with a 32-inch waistband seems about as likely as us owning a DeLorean car. We don't go out as much as we used to; in fact, most of our weekends are just repetitions of the same old thing. Does this sound a little familiar? Have you allowed yourself to settle into the metaphorical slippers and cardigan of middle age a little too early? Is the summer drone of your lawnmower more familiar to you than your favourite band?

I often ask myself the same question: 'Are you adding *life* to your days, or days to your life?' And when it's days that I'm adding, I close my eyes, have a quiet moment and think about something that I'd like to do which would give me excitement and be something to look forward to. And if it involves a little bit of risk, that's even better.

Until we take stock of ourselves and make changes, one day can seem much like another and, depressingly, it can feel as if we're just stacking time. When middle-aged men's lives become a predictable treadmill, they start to die inside. In the West, we've fallen into the trap of playing slavishly safe, following the trodden path of what we think is expected of us. Then we wonder why, a few decades down the line, life feels unsatisfactory and we are unhappy. Middle age spread in your fifties seems to appear just by even thinking of a beer and curry. Spiritually, something else is happening to many of us, as we feel ourselves getting nostalgic for our younger years. Then we start thinking it's all over now, and that we're halfway down a steep, 'no coming back from' slope that leads to the cemetery.

This kind of twisted thinking can drive us to take extreme measures. We start to notice everything about us which betrays our age: our fading hairline, our sagging chest muscles, the fact we get out of breath quicker than we used to, and that our our capacity to run up a broken escalator is not what it was. It's these little signs of mortality, not to mention hair now growing in nostrils and ears, and even on our backs, which start to convince us that physically we are on the slide. And this may go some way to explaining why a man might risk everything he's worked so hard to build and protect for a few moments of illicit pleasure. Because he's feeling old.

At the age of forty-nine, and on the cusp of the Big Fifty, I had an affair. I was about eight years into developing Parkinson's and deep into fertile ground for classic midlife unease; an online friendship with M, a girl I'd gone to school with deepened, and we fell in love with each other through our email letters.

The impact this wrong turn of mine had on my marriage and my kids was seismic. For one, I moved out of the family home, which killed me. Logistically, the new relationship couldn't work because she lived up north with two boys going through their GCSEs and A-levels, and I absolutely needed to be close to Aggs and Finn, so I couldn't move.

By now it was 2021. I was staying at my parent's house near Ludlow, an hour-and-a-half away (three hours on a round trip to Cirencester). Finny hadn't attended his sixth form college for a few months during his final year: he was too depressed, a direct consequence of my actions. He had lost his Heracles, and now there was just an empty space where my statue had once stood on the plinth of his estimations. It must have taken superhuman strength to pick himself up and return to college. He was devastated about what had happened. I had been his best friend and the bottom of his world had fallen out. And I was equally devastated; Finn was my best friend, too, and I was now barely a ghost of my former self to him. Aggie dealt with it by putting me in a box, and in her presence no one could talk about me. It was as if I was dead.

Once the woman and I split up – by mutual agreement – Finny and I then had a chance to mend things. Seven months earlier, and before we came to Skye, I was still with her and took my son to see Jon Hopkins, the electronica artist, play live in Berlin. It was too soon after the split with his mum, but we still enjoyed each other's company. Finn witnessed how bad my illness now was; I was so Parky tired I could barely walk down the street, and my sweats were also constant. As for the dyskinesia, it was off the charts, and I was getting funny looks from people because of my involuntary movements. I was in pieces. One night, over dinner, the business of my leaving reared its ugly head and Finn revealed just how it had impacted on him, his mum and Aggie. I felt consumed with regret. What the hell had I been playing at? I sobbed with guilt in front of him. He didn't come over to comfort me; he was still too angry.

Thanks to the kids' mother, Ali, who believed our children needed to spend time with me regularly if they were to heal, I managed to see Finn and Aggs once during the week and at the weekend, when I would take my son out for driving lessons. The old Saab 900 wasn't the easiest car to learn to drive in, as it was huge, heavy and unwieldy, not to mention very fast, but we would have the roof down, Bowie playing on the sound system and Finn at the wheel. On a sunny day I'd take Aggs for a drive, with her and I catching the wind in our hair as we drove with the windows down, which she found very exhilarating.

What I did still fills me with regret. Ever since, I have done my best always to be there for my kids and to keep letting them know how much I love them. I've also built a reasonably good relationship with their mother, not just by financially looking after them as best as I can, but by trying to forge a new friendship with her based on honesty, respect and optimism, and on moving forward. Because of our kids, Ali and I will always be tied together, so it makes sense for us to be as civil as we can. Also, I'm very lucky because she is a fine mother; the best.

What is it that makes middle-aged men reach out and grasp at something for which we must pay a price bigger than we realise? What is it that attacks a man's judgment to the point that he would risk no longer being a part of the family he has tried so hard to build with love and care? I think it's more than just a strong sexual call. A midlife affair is ultimately a last chance saloon for the ego, stamping down its authority in the face of old age.

It was 2019 when I first went to Skye in search of some cold water therapy. How time flies; I had now been wild swimming for a good five years. Rha Falls reminded me a little of Lothlórien, the great forest of the elves in *The Lord of the Rings*. It had a magic all of its own in the way sunlight fell in shafts and caught blobs of water falling in the cascade, turning them into mobile rainbows. The canopy was a ragged patchwork of copper leaves still yet to fall, broken by windows of blue sky. It was markedly warmer than most pools in Skye and I drifted on my back, listening to the thunder of the falls with my eyes shut. There was something fey and magnetic about this pool; it held you in its thrall. It gave me a sense of hope and, despite its opaque waters, as I looked down into the abyss, it seemed to clear the sad thoughts from my mind and grant me the clarity I needed to get on with my life and rebuild those special relationships that I had disrupted.

Chapter 6

Fairy Glen

Reconnecting

Finn and I had come to Skye for a week this visit, and he had the additional task of being the book's photographer and documentary maker. I often take pictures for my travel stories and sell them to newspapers, I have also written and shot a few books, but Finny has *naturally* a much better eye than me. I never tire of telling people he scored an A★ in his A Level Photography.

By now it was 2021, and Aggie could no longer move independently without the aid of a 'walker', essentially a frame with wheels and a little seat that gave her some support. Built as slim as an elf, she was, however, getting heavy and growing taller as any teenager, and because of the weakness in my right-hand side from Parky, I found it difficult to lift her. She, in turn, had little control over her body as it gradually slid down the sofa. So Ali was continually having to lift her up, which worried me, because if anything happened to Ali's back we were stuffed and I would have to move back in. Finn was a great help, but he wasn't always there; like any teenager he had his own life. He was so brilliant with his sister, knowing exactly what to do when she was frustrated or upset, that we called him 'the Aggie whisperer'. Each time I picked Aggie up, the bottom of my spine would scream in pain.

Communication with Aggs wasn't possible; she was restricted to using a thumbs up for 'yes', and thumbs down for 'no', so it was her eyes I looked at for her true expression. When she was little, she didn't talk a great deal despite the speech therapy, and by now the disease had robbed her of the ability to voice anything clearly. It became a guessing game, trying to understand what she was saying, and in the end, Aggs being Aggs, she chose the elegant way of not talking. I wondered what her teenage voice would actually sound like if she was given the chance to use it. I occasionally have dreams in which she can talk and we have long-ranging conversations about lots of things. The biotech company was making progress, but still it was a long way from any serious development, because of the red tape involved in the pharma sector, and millions of pounds were required just to keep the research going.

Finn and I coming to Skye together eight months after Berlin was another opportunity to mend our relationship, which, though no longer so fractured, still required work and communication. By bringing Finn to Skye and using his considerable talents as a documentary maker for this book, we got to spend more valuable time together.

Through helping him prep for his exams over the phone during the week, and cramming with him at the weekend, I had repaired some small part of the damage, but I still had to convince him I wasn't going anywhere again, and that my middle-aged madness was over for good. That was not done verbally, but just by being there for him and his sister.

It was already evening as we landed at Inverness, but the summer light was still in the sky. I was a bit taken aback when I saw my pal Matt; shorn of his dreadlocks, his full head of hair was now slicked back in curtains. He wore a smart green moleskin jacket and looked more like an eccentric country gent than a Viking. We gave each other a bear hug and I introduced him to Finn. I knew they would get on like a house on fire; both love music and both are cool characters who don't need to shout to be heard. They are equally laid-back. Indeed all three of us are.

With Matt at the wheel we cut through the Scottish Highlands in no time, and before we knew it we were on Skye, shooting over the Bifröst bridge, and passing Portree on our way to Uig in the far north. Matt delivered us safely to our base for the next six days, a B&B called Waterside House, run by a charming lady named Christine, the mother of Matt's great friend and fellow wild swimmer, Gordy.

She was instantly welcoming, like a character in a Brothers Grimm story, and showed Finn and I up to our bedroom, a cosy space with a well-positioned Velux window that looked out on to the harbour and nearby bay just over the road. It was spotless and homely. We had a special rate and a fine breakfast every morning to start us off.

As father and son, we had always been close, and a great deal of water had thankfully passed under the bridge since Berlin. I think Finn relished the opportunity to take the photos and spend time with his dad. Me, I couldn't have been happier.

That first evening at Waterside House, Matt wished us goodnight and said he'd be round at about 9 a.m, to pick us up the day *after* tomorrow, as some juicy clients had late booked for a wild swim tomorrow with his tour company, Soak up Skye. Finn and I were glad to have a day exploring together before we started work. Matt was staying at a friend's house, another wild swimmer called Matthew, whom I had met briefly for the first time at Glenbrittle Campsite, when Matt and I had climbed up to the mountain lake, Coire Lagan.

'Aren't there any men's wild swimming clubs in Skye?' I asked Matthew.

'Nah, just Gordy, me and Matt,' he said.

I remember that struck me as weird. What is it about men, especially in their fifties, that makes them not seek out each other's company? I love nothing more than going out with my old friends for a few beers and take great pride in my old friendships, but ask me to meet a bunch of strangers who are men or women and I can't be bothered. I wonder if I have always been like this. If you're being generous, you could say that perhaps it's a form of shyness, or else you could just say quite reasonably that I'm an unsociable bastard.

Who is that old boy? I ask my reflection most days.

That's you. I reply. *At least the shell of you. The real you is how you're feeling inside, not what you look like.*

At school, l I looked like a jock and I suppose for a time I was. For the school, I played squash and rugby, ran the 400m and swam. Like Marmite, I drew and repelled people towards me in equal measure. I was also a late creative, who at the age of seventeen discovered that I loved reading off-beat writers like Kerouac and Poe. In my final school year, the appeal of chasing after a wet rugby ball at training five times per week – as well as a game every Wednesday and Saturday – briefly lost its appeal when compared to sitting by a fan heater reading Laurie Lee's *As I Walked Out One Midsummer Morning* for the first time. I was a good rugby player, an aggressive ball winner and tackler, and was integral to the team. It was a given that I would play for the first team in my final year. And when I didn't turn up to training at the start of Michaelmas Term, all hell broke loose. I went my own way, feeling uncomfortable being part of an established elitist group. The upshot was that I had to go to the headmaster. I was the only pupil ever to resign from the first-team squad.

I hadn't intended to resign, for it to blow up like this, I just wanted to put the cat among the pigeons. Why, to what end? I still have no idea.

It became a *thing* and for a time I was kind of enemy number one with the teachers. I soon regretted it and missed playing. After about two weeks of not competing, I asked to play again, but the rugby master was true to his word and insisted I couldn't come back. I was like an exile. I was also vice captain of swimming, so was forced to do that instead. Looking back, I think I had to go through that sloughing off of a skin: I needed to feel like an outsider in order to find my voice and live an authentic version of myself. It just came at a price, losing my membership of the pack. Or of that particular pack. Every society needs outsiders, people that challenge the status quo: artists, writers, musicians, designers, cultural rebels. But these outsiders also need the company of society. They have their own crowd or tribe, because not to have one is to cease being human.

One thing I've realised as I've got older, is that this need for people is universal. We all need a tribe; people to play sports with, watch movies with, talk to, and friends we can trust utterly. A friend is as vital as the air that you breathe. A good one is a safe port in a storm, someone who understands you, and an objective observer who can take a step back and help you understand your actions. And a real friend pulls out the best of you, since for a decent friendship to flourish involves a fair deal of give and not just take. I much prefer listening to a friend's story or problem, than I do telling my own.

By the time we are fifty, we should have a pretty clear idea of who our friends are and hopefully have an understanding of the things that upset and drive us mad, but equally of what makes us happy too. Knowing this is essential. I know that I am fundamentally a kind, genuine and loyal person. I also understand that I am independent, stubborn, often late and disorganised. I'm also a brave individual who will take risks to save others, and I have to remember I am getting older. I am guilty of overthinking things, and sometimes I don't think at all. I am sensitive and also very occasionally, when pushed, have a volcanic temper. Which characteristics were with me at birth and which are the product of nurturing or experience? Who knows, or cares, but they all need taking care of now!

I believe we are all wired a certain way, and we are who we are at base level. Yet we are not finite but organic things, always becoming, always evolving, and it is up to us what we change into. Being more conscious of our actions and what energy we are putting out there is a start. And to do this it helps when you recognise certain behaviours which spring directly from your ego. The ego has been described as the veil between what you think you are and what you are. It relies on stories to big itself up, and can produce these fables as evidence in a flash. When I was boxing, it used to amuse me how diligent my ego was. When I was given a proper boxing lesson from a superior fighter, for a while I would crash back to earth and realise that I was a pretty average boxer and getting too old to be putting myself in harm's way. I'd probably feel like that for the whole weekend, but by the start of the next week I was dying to get in the ring again, my ego ready to convince me I was much better than I actually was!

And back when I was an actor, because my ego was so bruised by the constant rejections, I felt the need to talk about myself – about the job that I'd been for and was hoping to do, and some of the jobs I'd done – in a desperate bid to validate myself. This was the ego at work protecting me, or so I thought. When a friend landed a good acting gig, I would find it hard to be genuinely delighted for them, wishing that we had both won a role in the same series – or less charitably, I wished that just I had got it! I never much liked myself in the thirteen years I was an actor; the profession just didn't sit right with me. And my battered and bruised ego was given free rein to run my mental house, and it did so in its own particularly ugly way. I was more interested in me than anyone else.

Thank God for my kids. They've brought my life into balance, made me realise that there are much more important things to worry about than myself. I thank travel writing, too, as it made me realise the little place I lived in as an actor was not the whole world at all, but just a very small place where not a great deal went on. Please don't think I'm diminishing other actors, I'm just talking about just me here.

There are some very clear signs of when your ego is in the driving seat, and one of these is an inability to walk away from a conversation you just know is going to flare into an argument. You know how things are going to turn out and yet you still insist on being proved right at all costs. Another example of the ego at work is when you blame others when things go wrong, and are never accountable yourself. Or when you're constantly making assessments about other people. Are they better looking than you? Do they earn more money? Or do you feel threatened by their success? And there's probably a bit of *Schadenfreude* in there too, experiencing joy at another's misfortune. Do you feel like you're obsessed about winning? That's the difference between trying your best and wanting to win, and being plain overcompetitive.

Neuroplasticity is the process by which the brain can rewire itself, creating new neural pathways and synapses to adapt to damage in the brain. If the left-hand side of the brain, the part which controls speech gets damaged, the right side may pick up some of the slack to help. It's like a minor road that grows into a superhighway the more you focus on it with new habits and actions. For instance, as Parky has worsened, it has become harder to drive. Manual transmissions are just too complex, but in automatic cars I've learnt to control the car pedals with my left foot. It took a little while, but now it works brilliantly.

Bruce Lee was a master of neuroplasticity before anyone much had heard of the word. In 1969 he was in serious trouble after injuring his back during a routine training session. The problem was that he hadn't warmed up properly. He was told by doctors that he might never walk normally again, and could certainly forget about practising martial arts ever again. Not allowed to move from his bed for six months, for a time Lee allowed himself to be depressed and feel sorry for himself. It was as if he needed to work through these demons of doubt.

But then it occurred to him that he knew his body better than any doctor, and that there were no hard and fast rules beyond the doctors' dire prognoses. He could choose to listen to them or follow his own path. The room he was stuck in became less his jail and more his think-tank, library and laboratory. He was full of purpose, and his goal for the immediate future was simple and clear – to prove the doctors wrong and to walk properly again.

Lee read up on nutrition, kinesiology, biomechanics and yoga, basically anything that was going to contribute to him getting on his feet and walking again. Next, he started writing his affirmations and goals on the back of business cards and placed them on his bedroom wall so he would constantly notice them, and the first thing that he saw on the ceiling on opening his eyes was one of these. One of the core messages he seeded his imagination with was 'walk on'. He also wrote a letter to himself that read:

'I, personally, will be the highest-paid Oriental super-star in the United States. In return I will give the most exciting performances and render the best quality and the capacity of an actor. Starting in 1970 I will achieve world fame and from then onwards till the end of 1980 I will have in my possession $10 million. I will live the way I please and achieve harmony and happiness.'

Coming from a guy who wasn't even predicted to walk properly again, this might seem like a big ask. But Bruce Lee made this slow gruelling change possible by replacing his self-doubt with constant affirmations to himself as to why he was doing the strenuous exercises; to give him back the physical poise that he had tempo-rarily lost and by having a really clear vision of what he wanted to get to.

Lee would later write that 'with every adversity comes a blessing, because the shock acts as a reminder to oneself that we must not get stuck in routine'. He was convinced that we can heal ourselves through the way we think, stripping down negative thoughts and being self-aware of the mental diet we are feeding ourselves.

After a welcome lie-in our first morning in Skye, followed by an amazing full breakfast, Finn and I set out to walk the Fairy Glen; one of the most enchanting places I've ever seen. It's not a place that you go to wild swim, as there's only a rather forbidding peat pool there. From our guest house in Uig it was about an hour's walk through the Uig woods, past the Rha Falls, taking a left turn after the Uig Hotel, then on past the cemetery on the top of the hill and a bit of a tramp through the wild north of the Trotternish Peninsula.

Cars began to appear parked up at the side of the road as if left abandoned, and then it came into view, a strange otherworldly knob of rock which rises like a tower from the ground and trees that surround it. The world and his wife come here to climb it. It takes about five minutes' climbing, but by the time you're at the top it can be a bit vertigo inducing, as there are no rails to stop you plummeting to the ground far below. Around this fantastical natural formation are dotted rowan trees, adding to its charm.

But it's not only this weird basalt rock formation that leaps straight out of a trippy 1970s Athena poster. It's the land around it, as the glen is made up of small conical mounds that look like burial cairns, each one with a spiral pattern upon it. They look as if they are man-made or rather fairy-made, as they are seem far too small for humans, but in fact it was the elements which sculpted these bizarre creations 100,00 years ago ...

It was a perfect day to go walking and to chat, the weather baking hot with a merciful breeze to keep the midges at bay, the sky a rich denim colour. I wore a bandana on my head to stop me catching too much sun. Having explored the Fairy Glen and now doused in magic, we took a path less travelled from the valley and ended up in a wood that felt like nobody had entered for many years. Sunlight fought its way through the overhead hollows of vegetation, dappling dangerous-looking toadstools, fallen boughs necklaced in finely spun spiderwebs and gnarled trees that looked like anguished spirits. I felt just being here in Skye was making me better.

By the time we returned down to Uig harbour, the sun was westering into the ocean and it was time to eat. We sat in the pub restaurant by the harbour eating fresh mussels and fries. When we'd finished, we got a couple of beers and sat outside, watching the ferries come and go.

'Thanks for coming, son,' I said.

Finn smiled, 'Thanks for asking me.'

I felt like my insides were lit by the sun.

Chapter 7

The Marble Pools

Balancing Your Inner and Outer World

It was early summer 2023 and the island of Skye was thrumming with fireweed, cowslips, forget-me-nots and bright yellow broom which threw up the scent of vanilla. The sun was mellow on our cheeks in the early morning, but it didn't take long for a loose cohort of midges to seek us out as we made for the water.

Human beings are drawn towards the colours of aquamarine and turquoise like blood-fixated gnats to an over touristy spot. It is as if we are programmed to get all excited about these colours with a childish delight. And the more unexpectedly these gorgeous hues are threaded into the landscape, then all the better for that. In Skye, there are there are three different shades of waterfall: peat brown, clearwater and varying shades of turquoise. The Marble Pools are decidedly turquoise. Leaving the car parked on the road to Elgol, we padded across the boggy country to find them.

What colour will it be sir?
Gin clear, whiskey peat, bottle green, or turquoise?
Then climb in and the old isle of mist goes to work on you
with her ancient fingers.
But first she tests your mettle,
and if you can fight your way through her frozen thickets,
beyond lie all the treasures in her healing waters.

'How did you discover these pools, Matt?' I asked.

'If you do enough walking on this island, you become an unofficial dowser, it's like you just know where water is going to be. The first time I had a sense of these pools, I was sure there was something spectacular going on down below, I just wasn't sure what, as there was so much vegetation. Then as I got closer, I heard a raging torrent and I knew it was a waterfall, but one that was hidden.'

'So what did you do?'

'I made a mental note of where it was and I resolved to come back and check it out.'

What a fantastic way to spend your days, I thought to myself. Matt wasn't doing it for any reason other than because he liked walking on the island and discovering natural treasures to swim in. Did you need a stronger reason than that?

'But I never expected it to be so perfect. Here comes the first pool,' he added.

It must have been 20 feet long and a little slimmer in breadth. The pool was fed by a hollowed-out channel in the rock. I wondered what this pool had witnessed in its early days: perhaps dinosaurs and the passing of ice ages. It was exquisite, crafted by ancient gods at the beginning of time. The sun lit the water an electric green, and I was near hypnotised as I watched it flow down in a beautiful white cascade. And to mark the spot where the water fell, there was a heart-shaped rock underneath, quite different to the rest of the stones at the bottom. Completely smoothed out by the run of the water, it had become a sandy bowl that invited you to sit in it and be massaged by the gentle hands of the waterfall.

'I'm speechless,' I said, manually closing my mouth. 'Really, I don't think I've ever seen anything so beautiful in all my life.'

'There's more to come. Try to ignore these first two pools and experience them later, on the way back.' I did as I was told and tried very hard to not look through my fingers at the next pool – smaller and just as beautiful, but decidedly stiller – which appeared five minutes' walk further on. With the summer sun beating down on our backs, I just wanted to slide into it.

We were now climbing a little, having got changed at the first pool into dryrobe, shorts and booties. My dyskinesia was awful that day, my hands and arms suddenly reaching out spasmodically into the air for no reason, and on repeated occasions I nearly lost my footing on slippery rocks and went for a Burton. As ever, Matt and Finn took it in their stride and pretended not to notice.

As we followed the meanderings of the stream, which in places had almost dried up so you could see the naked river bed and its rich spectrum of different stones and pebbles, it took us through a stand of trees, and around a corner until we were within hearing distance of the water-fall. A narrow schism in the rock face admitted the intrepid traveller, and I could now see the purest water thundering down in a noisy torrent of the brightest turquoise. It looked like a Caribbean jungle scene in an old Bounty advert. You had to wade into it to reach the inner sanctum, and then the floor disappeared abruptly beneath you so you were treading water. There was a gallery directly behind the waterfall where you could sit, look up and see the water tumbling down in a powerful foamy white torrent, above it trees growing out of the rock face at weird angles. Like the three monkeys, we sat and shared the space with a very laid-back frog the size of my thumbnail who was so perfectly camouflaged I almost sat on him.

But this was the wrong space to sit still for a long time. It was almost as if it was impossible to chill here: instead, you wanted to flop around like salmon, diving under-water into the stunning pool, exploring the cut in the rock at the bottom which opened up to an underwater cave. It was a little bit of a *Boy's Own* heaven, with all the perfect ingredients: the colour of the water, the sheer drama of the place and the fact that it was so well hidden. You just knew that not that many people had ever savoured it before. There's something about swimming in turquoise water that approaches perfection for me, but it was the unexpectedness of this watery oasis that held me entranced.

The sun was still high in the sky when we moved, with great reluctance, away from Marble Pool One and made our way downstream to the second tier. The second pool had a distinctly different feel to its siblings. It was not fed by a cascade but rather a quiet stream, and it was shaded by the lee of a cliff from which a profusion of fern and twisting tree limbs sprouted. There was something about its stillness that invited the visitor to sit down on its baby smooth sides and meditate on the moment. Every body of water has its own energy, and this one was a sanctuary of silence and peace. The water here was bottle-green with splashes of turquoise. It was no larger than 15 feet in circumference and shaped like a tear. We climbed in. The sun was stronger now and the pool was quite shallow, which meant it was warmer and you could stay in for as long as you liked. And we stayed a long time.

After some idle chat, we each drifted to our inner chambers of thought and stayed there awhile. Personally, I was thinking about the effects that different waters seem to have on me; when I'm in still water I seem to be able to focus and calm my energy, and when I'm in moving water I feel much more kinetic with a need to 'do'.

Water has the ability to give us energy, but equally bestows a level of focus. While sitting in that tear-shaped pool of turquoise I found my mind calmly focusing on things that needed to be done back in England. It was not worry in any shape or form, but rather that my mind was at peace and ready to sort things out rather than run away from them.

As we towelled off and made for the final pool, I asked Finn and Matt where their minds had been in the last 5 or 10 minutes while sitting quietly still. Matt lit a roll-up. 'I don't know, but this pool seems to help you focus on things,' he said.

Finn added, 'I was thinking about doing an MA in film at the Met School in Berlin. I found that my thinking was really linear and I could stack up the building blocks leading to spending a year there, and how I was going to get my showreel ready, and save the money up.'

'Actually, I did think of something,' said Matt, 'I was thinking specifically about my sculpture exhibition and the next thing that I'm going to do with it.'

So all of us in fact had been thinking about something specific, and really focusing on in depth. And it was all down to the energy the pool possessed. It had directly influenced our mood and levels of vitality. We didn't stay much longer than an hour here, our human curiosity drove us on to witness the last pool. Again, there was an almost perfect sandy-coloured bowl that received the white water, whereas the rest of the pool was dazzling turquoise with the rays of the sun falling on the dark grey stone at its bottom. I wondered how these beautiful bowls, large enough for half a dozen people to sit in, had got there? Nature has a way of positioning things in just the right place. There was something so pleasing about sitting back in the pool and watching the white water fall down the natural groove of the rock into the cupola, the way it had done for thousands upon thousands of years. This moment in time was a mere a blink of an eyelid and my life represented such a short span of time in the process of this groove being steadily eroded by the stream upon the rock creating the channel. Yet even as a transient passer-by, I was a part of its story.

Once again, we were playful, diving underwater and swimming. It also got me thinking about introversion and extroversion and how, whether we're introvert or extrovert, it's still important to have more of people's company rather than less of it. If we spend a portion of our time deep thinking, that has to be bookended by the company of others. It's just like the still pool with a cascade on one side and the plunging pool on the other, because it is to others that we naturally belong, not to our own solitary company.

The Stoics believed in something called *sympatheia*, which basically means we are all children of the universe, tied to each other and infinitely connected. And irrespective of the colour of our skin and the diversity of our beliefs, we should realise that when our thoughts reach out to other people, it is then most of all that we feel a sense of our connection to others, and a deep association with the wider universe.

My natural capacity for enjoying my own company and reading and researching establishes me quite clearly on the introvert scale. This surprises me a little bit, because when I was growing up I was decidedly more extrovert, but as we have seen in this chapter, we are never still, but always subject to change and the flux of life. We are becoming, adapting, reacting and evolving.

Matt has lived in Skye now for eleven years. He and his wife Michelle had originally planned to move up to Edinburgh where he would continue his work as a sculptor. Michelle was a historian, and so the bright city seemed tailor-made for her. But en route, the magnetic Isle of Skye intervened and brought them here instead. 'Outdoor living taught us we needed so few things apart from a warm house and food,' Matt told me. 'We got ourselves outside, out into the cold air, got our bodies moving through walking. Skye also rewired our brains to what mattered most, and that was feeling happy. Also, I started going in the water more; lochs, rivers, they seemed to draw me to them.'

'Every day,' Matt says, 'I looked for something new, fresh directions to walk. One day I found a burn (large stream) on a map which just sort of stopped abruptly. I wondered if it contained pools or falls or none of the above. So I walked that burn and followed it upstream with deep banks and then cliffs on either side of me.'

'I knew crofters would never do this because they didn't have the time for leisure activities. And there are not many people like me on the island, as dogged and obsessive about finding new spots. So when I eventually found the five pools upstream, it was a lovely feeling, a vindication of my efforts. I was satisfied with my trailblazing and it was as if I'd discovered them, which made them mine. Like dowsing, I had just known that there would be pools upriver. I can almost smell them these days, and I can tell which rocks will make a good pool, so I can see it before it's even there. I think we are drawn to water. Just as water babies are drawn to one another's company.'

After the majesty of the Marble Pools, the following day we visit Carbost falls. The weather has turned, there's a grim sky above, and the air is cold and uninviting. Swimming in freezing cold water or even dipping do not sound like options I particularly warm to today. But as is almost always the case, when I see wild water it's as if my inner me knows just what good it will do if I *do* slip in and get wet. Carbost falls lights my heart on this dull day. With its steep fall and pure white cascade, plus the darkness of the basalt rock behind, it is one of the prettiest cascades I've ever seen. It's also very easy to reach; you'll find it located just half a mile south-west of the little village of Carbost. To get to it you'll need to climb over the barbed-wire fence if you're coming from the old Victorian school house and then follow the burn upriver a short way. It's possible to take the road that drives above the fall and look down on it, but if you're coming to swim you need to catch the former and park anywhere on the verge.

Apparently, just standing by a waterfall is like mild hypnosis and it raises your serotonin levels, as the fall is a natural source of negative ions; so the sound of crashing waves or the thunder of a cascade recharges our batteries and makes us feel great again. Our energy is made up of both positive and negative ions, and yes, it sounds a little arse-over-tit, but it is apparently positive ions which we get from computer screens and phones and also from being locked up indoors and constantly under artificial light. Whereas, ironically, it's the negative ions that are good for us. And while it's great to stand aside a beautiful double cascade whilst filling up your serotonin tanks, there is no substitute for being *in* the falls, your flesh bare.

I remember the time we were halfway up the mountain on the return journey from Camasunary Bay, and I passed a babbling brook which flowed under the track we were walking on. Just hearing and then glimpsing it moving purposely, seemed to give me some energy. Even the crabbiest person feels a change in their energy when they're standing beside a waterfall.

Once at Carbost Falls, we waste little time getting in the water. The rocks are slippery in the riverbed on our approach and the air has teeth today. A silver birch tree stands like a narrow-shouldered sentinel right beside the blue pool into which the 80-foot cascade drops its load. The water is cold and vital as we slowly lower ourselves into it. Finn, meanwhile, has become an ace with the drone camera in a very short space of time; it has almost become like a witch's familiar, always hovering above his shoulder! With their constant playing on Xbox and Nintendo games, his generation have developed such brilliant hand-to-eye coordination that it makes no difference whether Finn is controlling a real, tangible thing or an avatar on the screen. He's really grown into his role as a director on this shoot. Every shot has been storyboarded and planned, he works his film camera seamlessly and backs material up as soon as he can. He's learning the lesson of not trying to do too much on your own all at once. The one thing he does forget to say is 'Cut!', and Matt and I are left like a couple of partially dressed actors standing beside the waterfall awaiting direction.

Matt decides he is going to climb up the grass cliff next to the fall, and naturally I follow, despite my balance playing up that morning. Too often we think of what could go wrong instead of what can go right. I could have a fall, but what sense is there focusing on that when there are so many great things that can happen instead? I don't even let the doubts enter my mind. In no time we are up high, level with the fall on the grassy cliff. I find a comfy seat of ferns and, like some modern day Poseidon, I sit upon this throne and ponder the extraordinary view below and into the distance.

In a straight line from us the burn travels directly to the loch. There is a small window of blue where the sky is gazing through the rainclouds and I'm just beginning to relax into the landscape when a word I was trying to remember yesterday in a pub in Portree comes back to me: '*Friluftsliv*' (pronounced *free-loofts-liv*). It's funny how things come back to you at the most unlikely time!

Friluftsliv is a Scandinavian term, which, literally translates as 'free-air living', and describes the spiritual benefits of spending time in forests, wild water and remote places. It's basically immersion in natural places, but with it comes a kind of self-healing and reverence for being outside in the great outdoors. I remember my Norwegian friend Egil, whose son Noah started school at the age of six, and who for first couple of years learned forestry skills and spent most of the time outside before he even went near a textbook. In Norway, the average toddler at nursery school spends up to 80 per cent of their time in the summer months outside. And because of this a bond between man and nature has already been developed in the child early on. Subconsciously, the blueprint for a happy balanced life involves getting outdoors whatever the weather, every day, and connecting with it. *Friluftsliv* is a very real strand of *sympatheia*, of being in touch with that bigger picture in which we realise we are all responsible for the caretaking of this planet and are deeply linked to one another. It's about respecting and generating positive energy from nature.

As I remember this, a sense of wellbeing washes over me. That and gratitude. Wild swimming in these waters

Swimming with the Viking of Skye at the 'Circe's eye' pool, Loch Coruisk.

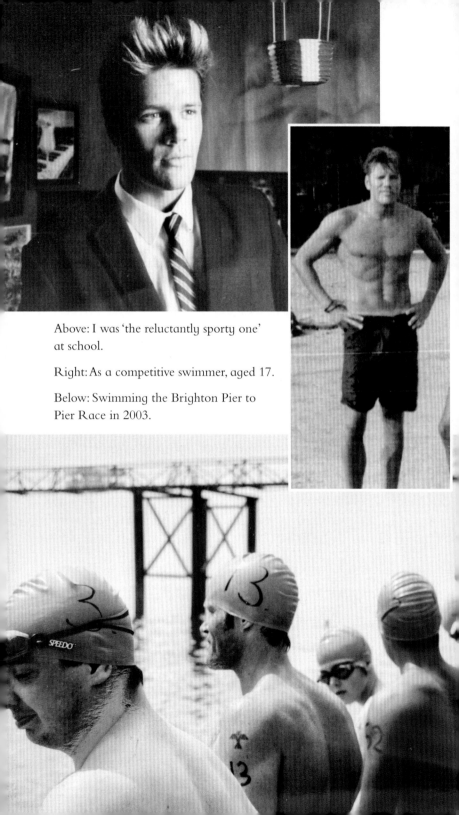

Above: I was 'the reluctantly sporty one' at school.

Right: As a competitive swimmer, aged 17.

Below: Swimming the Brighton Pier to Pier Race in 2003.

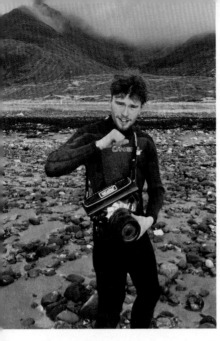

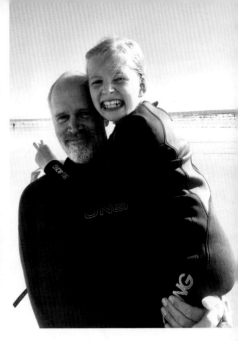

Above left: Finn at Camasunary Bay.

Above right: Aggie and Dad, Saunton, Devon, 2018.

Below: Half way up to Coire Lagan. 'The harder it is to reach, the wilder the swimming.'

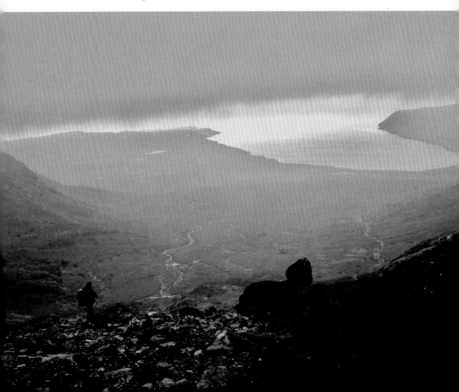

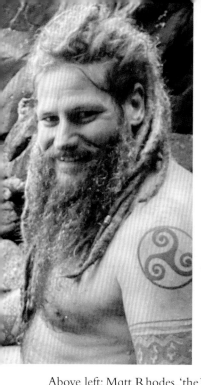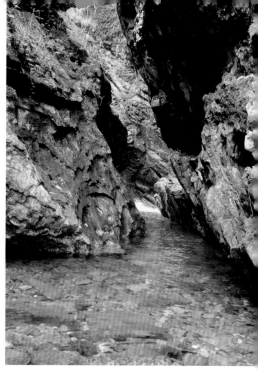

Above left: Matt Rhodes, 'the Viking of Skye'.

Above right: The final route to the Marble Pool cascades, Pool One.

Below: With ex-Special Forces Soldier Ollie Ollerton.

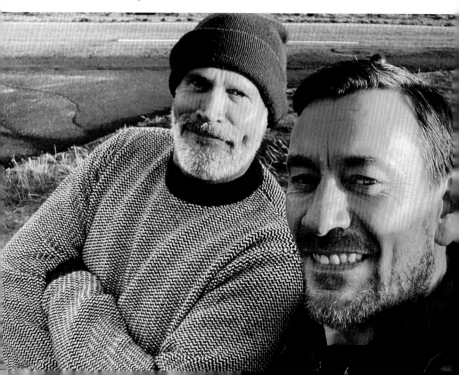

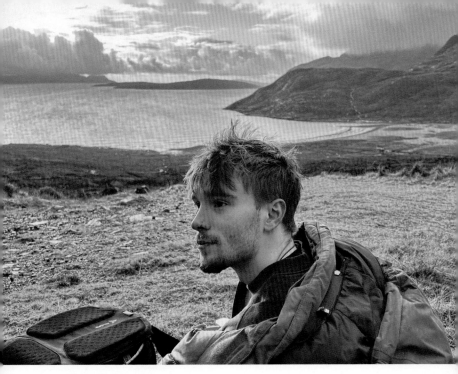

Above: Finn at Camasunary Bay.

Below left: Inside Flodigarry Sea Cave.

Below right: At the entrance to the cave.

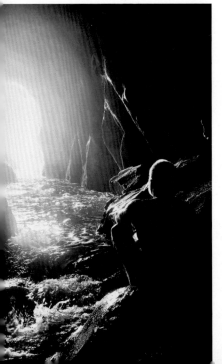

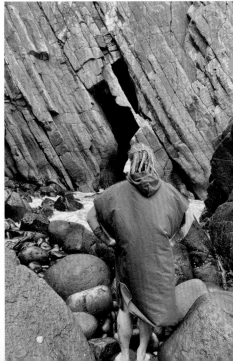

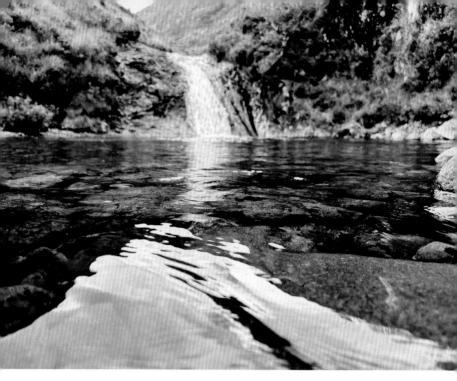

Above: Marble Pool Two.

Below left: Matt rising to the surface of the Healing Pool.

Below right: Matt at Marble Pool Two.

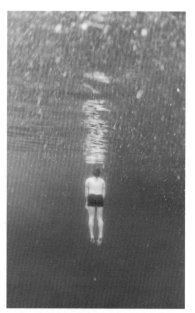

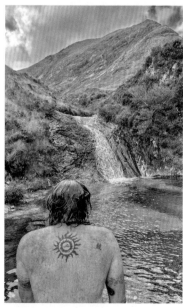

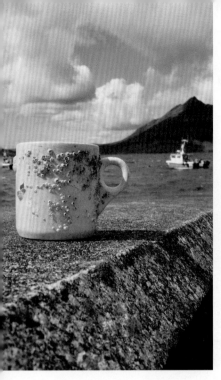
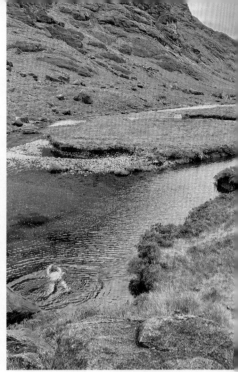

Above left: The quay at Elgol, the departure point for Loch Coruisk.

Above right: Matt in the 'Circe's eye' pool at the end of Loch Coruisk.

Below: Matt at the Healing Pool.

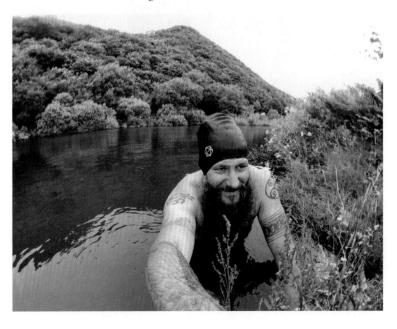

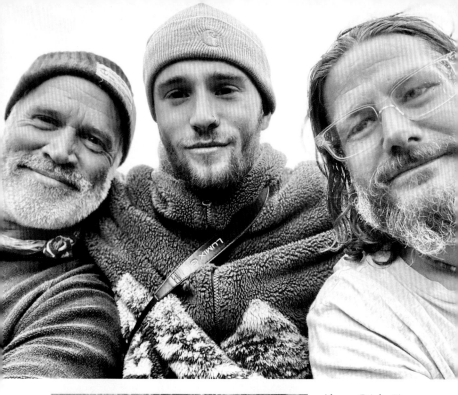

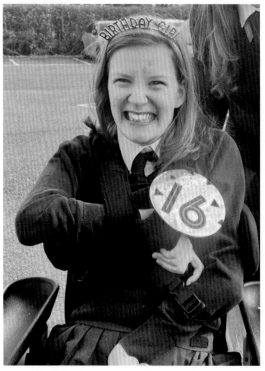

Above: Rich, Finn and Matt en route to Coruisk.

Left: Aggie, aged 16.

doesn't just feel good, it's a tool for gaining personal insights and improved wellbeing. It makes me notice things in a more pronounced way. After I've been wild swimming, colours pop where I would usually not notice them: I look into people's eyes more curiously and notice they aren't just blue but flecked with other colours, too; I notice their expressions because I want to reach out and connect with them. Also, I am more relaxed in myself and I feel more generous. Not a bad dividend for climbing in a freezing cold pool in a pair of trunks!

Chapter 8

Loch Shianta,
the Healing Pool

Be Done with Self-Loathing

When we wake up in the morning our mind is free of negative self-talk for probably less than a minute. And then as we lie there, coming to and shrugging off the vestiges of sleep, those self-sabotaging thoughts start firing at us like darts. Meanwhile, our inner critic is already wittering on in our ear, presenting us with pessimistic reminders of things that may go wrong this new day, and perhaps what went wrong yesterday. If we listen to this critic, we'll start the day on the wrong foot, but if we develop an understanding of where that inner critic is coming from and why, we can learn to sidestep it and avoid the anxiety it creates.

An estimated 60,000 thoughts go through our head every day and about 90 per cent of them are unconscious repetitions of those we had yesterday, which are in turn themselves echoes from those of the day before. And so on.

We live in an echo chamber of repetition. Our brain has the tireless task of constantly trying to make sense of the world around us. In order to save time and brainpower and not be constantly overwhelmed by new stimuli or unfamiliar situations that present themselves to us, our mind does a rapid sort of Google search in our 'unconscious hard-drive' and returns a millisecond later with a suggested response, based on similar situations we've already experienced. This is your computer mind being lazy, and it's often way off the mark, which is why we can get disproportionately defensive or angry with people when we misunderstand them. It's because we've been given the wrong instructions by our brain.

What, you might ask, does your brain do if there's nothing remotely similar in our memory to the situation we currently find ourselves in. What happens then is that a mental panic button is automatically pressed and we switch into emergency mode (otherwise known as fight or flight). Often, there is nothing to be scared about, it's just the ancient part of our brain on high alert because it thinks that this unknown scenario could spell danger.

When we observe our thoughts, rather than get swept up in them, we begin to understand our mind more and recognise unhelpful trains of thought. Learning to be an observer of yourself allows you some distance from your instinctual behaviour. The next time you see red or feel a sense of panic which is not proportionate to the situation, try and step outside yourself and notice old opinions surfacing, or unjustifiably negative self-talk. Unless we monitor the thoughts which are creating *feelings* in us from moment to moment, there's every chance that we will be feeding ourselves negative thoughts that keep bringing us down.

Ever since leaving the family home, I had been burdened with terrible guilt and self-loathing. I had not only broken a personal code of ethics by leaving, I had also broken the hearts of my children, despite they being more important to me than anything else. I couldn't stay with Ali any longer for obvious reasons, but I didn't want to leave my girl and boy. It was an impossible situation.

Unless I could start to respect myself again and forgive my fractured psyche, I would be forever condemned to this state of self-loathing. One of my best friends is an alcoholic. Sober now for some twenty-nine years, he has some of the most brilliantly helpful phrases of wisdom that he pulls out of his pocket when I most need them. One day, hearing me repeat my self-hating mantra for the umpteenth time, about how I had fucked my life up and the people I most loved, he told me the serenity prayer, 'God grant me the serenity to accept those things which I cannot change, the courage to change that which I can, and the wisdom to know the difference.'

With that in mind, I couldn't change what I'd done but I could certainly ensure it never happened again. The first step toward healing was to try my best to win back the trust of those whom I'd let down. Actions speak louder than words when somebody has lost confidence in what you say. It might take a long time, and things might never again be the same as before, but I was prepared to do anything.

We may experience life through our feelings, but it is our thinking which initiates these feelings in the first place. The relationship we have with ourselves dictates the level of happiness in our life. If you think uncharitably about yourself, this will be reflected in everything you do; from the way you talk to others to how you allow others to talk to you. Your sense of self-worth colours the way you respond to every situation you come across in life, and if you don't *think* you're worthy of luck, love, esteem and success, you will forever be people-pleasing, aiming low and letting others walk over you. Continually being penitent wasn't going to solve anything for me. I needed to remind myself of some of the good things that I had achieved in life, and so I began to list times when I had helped other people. It went back as far as primary school, where I stood up to the school bully to protect another little four-year-old kid. And from then on, I had always fought the corner of people weaker than myself. Later, as a journalist writing environmental pieces on wildlife, I was sticking up for animals where I could.

If you're suffering self-esteem issues, your journey towards equilibrium must start with becoming a better coach to yourself. You can't keep whipping yourself for the same crime; at some point you have to admit that you've served your time. It's an insult against nature for you to carry on wasting every precious day drowned in regret and self-contempt. It's about believing that, as a child of the universe, you have a right to be here. Marcus Aurelius once said, 'the soul becomes dyed with the colour of its thoughts'. And, stained with self-loathing, my thinking constantly tried to get me down. You can't wear this type of invisible horsehair shirt forever, and at some point you have to say, 'I've done my penance, and from here on I'm going to try and be the best version of myself. I *will* take accountability for my actions, every one of which has a consequence. I acknowledge what I've done and admit that it was wrong.'

I have been lucky enough to have been treated by the same neurologist for the last six years, and under Dr Alan Whone's compassionate care I have been able to better understand the machinations of this twisted and horrible disease. I had not seen him at the Bristol Brain Centre for the best part of a year, during which time my marriage had gone under. When I relayed to him what had happened, he was enormously empathetic and offered to call my wife and have a chat with her on my behalf. 'That's very kind of you,' I said, 'but I doubt there's much you can do.' My wife wasn't interested in hearing any scientific explanation; as far as she was concerned I was 100 per cent responsible for what I had done.

'What's happened with you is fairly common, and there's a reason for this,' he said, smiling at me sympathetically. 'Basically, the frontal cortex of your brain is the part which is responsible for rational thinking and it controls impulses, and makes you consider the consequences that can follow certain risky acts. People with Parkinson's have a diminished sense of consequence, because their frontal cortex is under attack from the disease. So, while in the past, for things that you might've wanted to do but knew you shouldn't, you had a natural brake to stop you following that temptation. This you no longer have, and as a result you can get yourself in some pretty tight situations.'

There were lots of things to be hopeful about. I wasn't a bad person, just somebody who had made some crappy decisions without the aid of a working frontal cortex and was now paying for it. We live most of our life inside our heads in our thoughts, so why should I make it a place which was wallpapered in remorse? I had to try and get on with life and start healing from the inside. I needed to start turning that hideous wallpaper which was cartooned with my faults, into sunny faces and sunbeams. Bruce Lee is often quoted as saying, 'Don't speak negatively about yourself, even as a joke. Your body doesn't know the difference. Words are energy and cast spells, that is why it's called *spelling*. Change the way you speak about yourself and you can change your life. What you're not changing you're also choosing.'

It was overcast as Matt and I drove to the north of the island. My mind was a bit like the weather. The Trotternish Peninsula is an other-worldly place of giant black basalt cliffs the octagonal shape of church organ pipes, and was formed in the Jurassic era 150 million years ago. As we drew closer to a huddle of giant spear-like rocks to the west of us, I noticed a colossal column of basalt standing out independently from the other formations.

Matt caught my eye. 'Look familiar?' he asked.

'It does, very. Why do I think I've seen it before?'

'It's at the start of *The Wicker Man*. You know, that creepy old film about pagan magic.'

My face must have lit up, 'You serious? That's one of my favourite films!'

'That needle of rock is called the Old Man of Storr, and it's in the titles at the start of the film, when the policeman – played by Edward Woodward – is flying his seaplane over it as he heads to Summerisle to investigate a young girl's disappearance.'

'I remember it."

'Local lore says it's the penis of a giant who fell and was covered by the earth.'

We chatted as the rain beat an incessant drumbeat on the roof of his car. 'Geek alert, but did you know that they filmed *The Wicker Man* to look like summer,' I said, 'but it was actually the dead of winter, and all the blossom for the trees had to be brought in and stuck, flower by flower, to the branches.'

'You're joking.'

'And those naked women dancing around the fire in the ring of stones? They were so cold they had to wear skin-coloured body suits.'

'Nice.'

Only another fellow film nerd would appreciate this. Again, my mind returned to the theme of guilt; unlike the selkies – mythical figures who could choose the form of either the seal or, on a moonlit night. remove their sealskin and become beautiful women – I couldn't just shake this penitent skin off me. Plagued, like most of us are, by an inner police man excellent at pulling me down, it would take more than the bloody moonlight to slough it off.

Matt pulled into a car park on an incline, where a sign read: 'Loch Shianta, The Enchanted Holy and Magical Loch'. I didn't care how magical it was, I didn't much feel like climbing into freezing cold water today. The rain had finally ceased, and there seemed a chance the sun might break through.

'The islanders used to call it the "Lourdes of the North" back in the day,' said Matt. 'It's supposed to have healing power.'

To reach the healing pool, we passed through a little wood of trees forming a natural hollow with their withered outstretched branches. We had on our flannel dryrobes in readiness for a dip. Leaving the wood behind and rounding a corner, the path cut through a glorious green meadow of tussocky grass. As if to manage my expectations, Matt said, 'You might find yourself underwhelmed when you first spot it, but the closer you get ...' he smiled, 'Well, you'll see.'

I had noticed that Matt had a habit of not getting over-excited and not getting you over-excited, even about something which warranted it, like the pear-shaped pool with bottle-green water which soon appeared in the distance. Rather, he might be a little circumspect about its virtues. Not having overly great expectations is a very Stoic thing, and that way you're never really disappointed. But wasn't it Dr Johnson who once said, and I paraphrase, 'The expectation of an event is often superior to the event itself'? In other words, the looking forward to, and the getting excited about, is all part of the journey. I know that I am very much in this second camp and I find it hard not to get excited about certain things. A friend once said, it's a question of making your future as big as possible, because when you make your future busy you give yourself something to look forward to, and it reminds you in the present that you are doing something right and making the most of your life. I agree with this completely.

The pool was banked on one side by hazel trees. Matt wasn't wrong; the closer I got to the water, the more I picked up on its presence; it was as if it was drawing me inexorably towards it. When we were a few feet away and

I could look properly into its depths, I actually lost my breath. The bottom was made of sand and the sun, when it came peeping out of the clouds for an instant, lit the pool a rare emerald scattered with shots of turquoise, the shells at the bottom glittering like mother-of-pearl. It glowed with the sanctity of a stained-glass window in a church. I had to get in!

'You might want to take your time getting in mate,' Matt cautioned, 'this is one of the coldest bodies of water on the whole island. Holds its temperature at around 7–8 degrees, even in summer, because it's fed by a freezing spring that comes through the mountain.'

Using Matt's rule of thirds – that's to say gradually immersing yourself in three stages, the first being up to your knees, then to your waist and finally up to your shoulders and head, all so as not to traumatise your heart – I dipped my toe into the water and it instantly felt like it had just been bitten off!

'Shit, that's *cold*!'

It wasn't just the extreme low temperature that distinguished it from other pools we'd so far swum in. There was something 'special about this water, as if I could feel an infusion of wellbeing soaking into my skin, a fresh beginning, a clearing of the slate. Even the hardiest person would not last long in this water. When wild swimming, you have to listen closely to your body; on first contact with the cold water your fight and flight reflex will go into overdrive and try and make you get the hell out, but once you've got through this natural panic, you'll be fine. It's the next stage of cold you must be mindful of, and pushing back against your body's inner wisdom then will earn you a dose of hypothermia if you're not careful. If you're swimming in extremely cold temperatures, it's a question of acclimatisation by increments; not one huge statement, rather a series of smaller ones.

Once I had got used to the icy teeth biting at my naked flesh and relaxed my breathing, I swan-dived to the bottom, the depths skittering with sunshine in columns of twisting light. It was much deeper than I'd anticipated; I half expected to see a selkie swim towards me out of the murk. The water was enchanted. For a few seconds it was as if I was transported to an ancient place of magic and paganism. When I rose, breathless, to the surface, my body was on fire. My blood raced to my extremities to warm me up; every pore on my body tingling with glee. I had never felt so rejuvenated. As I towelled off and hurriedly threw a dryrobe over my body, I noticed the tremor had gone in my right hand; it was now completely still, and my dyskinesia was momentarily banished, giving me a few minutes' peace. And that unhappiness I was carrying around because of my shame had disappeared, at least for the time being.

'Long ago,' said Matt, 'the people who visited the pool weren't just locals, they came from all over, many of them mystics. They'd drink some of its water and make an offering of coloured thread. And even though there was trout in the pool, nobody would ever take any out. Nor would they cut any wood out of respect and fear of the place.'

'It does feel otherworldly,' I said, staring at the opacity of the water, trying to articulate what I had just experienced. 'At the bottom just now, I felt that if I was to swim into the dark bits of the pool in the shadow of the hazel trees, that there might be a kind of portal between this world and the next dimension, where the divide was somehow very thin.' Then I said, embarrassed, 'Listen to me talking utter bollocks!'

'Not at all mate, everybody gets different things from the pool. I'm not one for believing in the paranormal, but I admit, the place does have an energy all of its own.'

'I'm surprised that there aren't more people here,' I said.

'Luckily for us, it's pretty well hidden. And it doesn't do any harm that the locals often hide the sign to protect the place from being overrun. Unlike other sacred pools, this one is free of cloth scraps and coin offerings.'

'You mean like the Fairy Pools?' I asked.

'Exactly. The Fairy Pools became overrun with tourists a while back,' said Matt. 'Because the tourist board, council or whoever didn't control the numbers going there, and tourists' constant footsteps wore the paths that run beside the pools completely smooth.'

'So the place became a victim of its own success?'

'It gets worse. When it rains the path becomes lethally slippery. One guy fell in and had a heart attack because his body went into shock in the cold water. They've improved the paths now and built a bridge.'

Nobody else can heal you apart from yourself, and that must begin with reframing the way that you look at yourself. When you start self-caring through simple nourishing routines like shaving, taking regular exercise, sleeping and eating well, you feel like you are more in control of yourself and consciously start steering your thoughts in a positive direction. That's when good things start to happen, doors previously unseen or locked begin to open for you, and the more you listen to the space between your thoughts and breath, and trust, allowing yourself to just be, the more insights seem to come from your gut.

The mind is like a car windscreen and gets so clouded with a myriad of repetitive negative thoughts, that often you can no longer think or see clearly. Imagine that your chosen weapon to counter these thoughts – be it medi- tation or cold water swimming – is a windscreen wiper swishing the glass clean from one side to the other to allow a moment's clear view. This briefly lived clarity is your present, the place where insights can form and natu- rally flow towards you. I found that I was able to access this peace, a place free from thought, only when I was in the water and for a short time afterwards. And it was here in this freezing water that I began to heal.

The mind is a fuggy tool. *Fuggy*. Did I invent that word just now? For the record, by 'fuggy' I mean sometimes it's unreliable with the data it brings back. For instance, have you ever experienced an immediate dislike of a stranger or found yourself naturally gravitating towards one? There's a feeling in your gut, an instinct which is telling you, 'Watch out for this person they could be a threat!' Or, 'You can trust this person.' That's *fugginess*.

The reason that we often forget people's names when we are first introduced to them is because, as we are looking in their eyes, the brain is scanning their expression and posture to measure the level of threat that they might present. It's really that primitive. That's why first impressions are so powerful. If, having performed its scan, the brain comes back with nothing threatening to associate to this person we are seeing or meeting for the first time, it's business as usual and all is well. But if in its quick search of our memory it finds somebody similar – be they good or bad – it hands that over to the lizard part of the brain whose job it is to kick us in to fight or flight. That is why we experience the same feelings we did towards people dredged up from the past, transferring those to the perfect strangers before us. This is called 'the horns and halo effect' and illustrates how powerful our unconscious thoughts are and how misplaced they can sometimes be.

I can think of a few occasions when for no apparent reason I have had ill feeling towards perfect strangers; like when I saw *Dragons' Den* for the first time, and took an immediate dislike to one of the dragons who made me feel uncomfortable. I later realised that this was because my brain was confusing him with a brilliant boxer I'd forgotten about who, years earlier, had regularly given me a boxing lesson each time I stepped in the ring with him (and black eyes to boot). Then there was the new boyfriend of a friend of my wife's who I had a natural empathy with and felt like I knew him immediately. To be fair, he was a nice bloke in his own right, but without my realising it he reminded me of my favourite rugby coach at school, for whom I had had a great deal of respect.

Given that the brain is crap at cross-referencing and is often on autopilot, this explains why old unhelpful thinking goes unchallenged, and why we repeat our actions day in day out, even if they're not constructive in leading to a happy life and they fail to provide us with a decent opinion of ourselves. If the brain is recycling old thoughts which then dredge up old negative feelings, then you're going to end up living with recycled negative emotions. The better you get at observing yourself and the skin you're in, the quicker you'll get to work out what makes you tick and the bad stuff that makes you stuck.

So, now that we're all agreed our brain is unreliable and our thoughts are anything but 100 per cent accurate, it's not too much of a stretch to believe that we can filter our thoughts and change the messages we're giving ourselves, is it? We're not exactly the finished article. Well, I'm certainly not.

On a macro level, human brains are still evolving, but are made up of three main sections, each with a different job description. The lizard brain (aka the brainstem) is the dark primal pool where your instinctive behaviours spring from. It controls your breathing and heart rate, when you feel fear, hunger and anxiety; as well as pain, touch, smell, thirst, sexual urge and tells you when to sleep and wake. The lizard brain is the oldest part of the brain and is responsible for keeping you alive. If it sees fit, it will take charge of the horse brain and the human brain and shut them down temporarily to achieve survival.

In many ways, the lizard brain is an overreactor, unsuitable for today's times. Just think about it: we're too highly charged for our environment – look at the current levels of anxiety in our society. I find it weird to think that only 15,000 years ago we were still being hunted by bigger creatures than us with much sharper teeth. Maybe evolution needs a little longer to catch up and make us act less like frightened children always on the lookout for constant trouble.

The horse brain is our emotional centre where our urge to care for others and be cared for comes from. Love, hate, jealousy, pride and happiness, they're all governed from here. The horse brain is also where we store old and new memories which are used to tell us how to act in social situations, and how to respond emotionally to smells. It's also where motivation and purpose live, which is why when we are emotionally invested in something, we put our heart into it.

Finally, the most recent addition to our complex neural make up, is the human brain, the neocortex; home to rational thought, creativity, imagination and also responsible for trying to reason with natural impulses. When we're out on the town, drink too much alcohol and suddenly need to visit the men's room, it's the human brain that politely persuades our lizard brain not to unzip and relieve ourselves in the middle of the bar. With its pull towards patience and common sense, the neocortex is responsible for some of the greatest achievements of mankind, from the pyramids to the first dictionary.

Imagine the thoughts continually racing through your mind at any one time; these three brains have to decide what the right reaction is in response to them. No wonder the brain cuts corners to save us time. And it's this corner-cutting that we can play to our advantage. People who suffer depression produce less dopamine, and it is dopamine which reduces the stress chemical we produce called cortisol. When we exercise, we feel instantly better because it lowers cortisol levels and forces us to create dopamine, which not only helps us be more alert and engaged, it helps us be happier, and when we smile we release yet *more* dopamine.

Here is a trick with an immediate benefit, and it also goes to show how easy it is to consciously fool your brain. When you smile, a series of muscles and nerve endings in your cheeks align, and signal to the brain that you're happy; it then sends you a hit of dopamine to continue feeling like this. So, if you feel fed up and stressed, make yourself smile. You'll feel like you've lost your marbles but keep doing it – as your brain doesn't know the difference and sends the dopamine anyway. In other words, it's possible to trick ourselves into feeling better. And before we know it, we *do* feel genuinely better. And from this positive place we can continue making positives. TIP: hold a pen between your teeth, which will make you smile.

I was reading a lot of pop psychology, trying to find ways to trick my mind into being positive, as it took only a few moments ruminating on Aggie or myself to feel defeated, deflated and vulnerable to spiralling down. The other reason I was reading a lot of psychology was I'd taken on a new client as a co-author, and the book we'd write together would be a self-help book. His name was Tyson Fury.

It's very hard to be and stay in love if you're not loving yourself. And by that I don't mean constantly looking in the mirror and admiring yourself, I just mean having a strong level of self-respect. When you doubt yourself, you become a shade of yourself. This then affects your behaviour, and you can become more needy towards your partner without realising it. It's like a set of scales that once enjoyed an equilibrium, but which become stilted and overweighted on one side.

I had to get a grip, start exercising regularly, begin writing a journal and keep on top of work, writing a stipulated amount of words every day, calling friends regularly and generally marshalling my life. Once you start feeling more in control because you are consciously steering your thoughts in a positive direction, the more insights seem to come from your gut and the more you start to listen to the space between your thoughts and breath. I think it's about sending constant reminders of encouragement to yourself and being a good self-coach.

Tyson is a prime example of someone who can get swamped in negative thoughts and lose his sense of purpose. Thankfully, he rediscovered his mojo through a tough and consistent regimen of exercise, and that's what that book is about. During the pandemic, as we wrote the book together, another thing which massively helped him was sharing his exercise with a loyal band of followers online. In other words, he became part of something bigger than himself and his inner turmoil was put to one side so as to focus on others. He and his wife Paris never missed a day in which they weren't helping other people keep their sanity by doing something as simple as half an hour's exercise with kettle bells, press-ups or sit-ups, which they did – with constant interruptions from their kids – beamed live from their front room. It is so much healthier to put your focus on helping other people rather than on your own depression.

It was while writing this book with Tyson that I started following an acronym I created. I find it a really helpful way of incorporating a number of disciplines which soon become daily habits and you look forward to doing. They also keep you out of trouble. So, the acronym I chose was SHINE, and it stood for:

- Smoothie (one healthy fruit drink each morning)
- Hydration (drinking loads of water)
- Intention (for the day: e.g. 'today I will be a good listener to others')
- Nutrition (five a day)
- Exercise (swimming or running)

Establishing simple nourishing routines like taking regular exercise, eating well and positive self-talk are all really useful ways of feeling better. Remember, the mind is like a moving window. It will get clouded with thoughts which are repetitive and negative, they will come at you from both sides and the window will be continually fogged. Self-esteem is based entirely on *judgments*, whether from others or from ourselves. Yes, we need to feel good about ourselves. However, the answer is not to be found in what we do, what we say, how we look, how we perform and what others believe (though I believe in order to maintain self-respect we have to try our best at what we do and to take a sense of pride in it).

When we base our worth and love for ourselves on anything *external*, we will always fail. Basing our worth on our emotions can never succeed either, because those emotions are sometimes wrong or false, and at best they're bloody unreliable. We are more than how we feel about ourselves. Self-evaluation, too, can be a useful tool for personal growth, but we shouldn't base our *worth* on our thoughts and others' evaluations of us. But the problem with self-evaluation is we don't just compare ourselves to the progress we've made, we compare it to others and this is where we fall down.

My recovery, given the way I felt about myself, wasn't going to happen overnight. But this is where I struggled: 'How can I buy into this business of self-growth when another part of me is dysfunctional and gradually dying?' I asked myself.

And then I re-remembered Marcus Aurelius' statement about death – 'Think of yourself as dead. You have lived your life. Now take what's left of it and live it properly – that what doesn't transmit light creates its own darkness.'

My recovery lay in the present tense, not the future. I wanted to be honest, happy and fulfilled with the time I had left; it might be five years, at a stretch it could be ten. The self-worth a person feels is a deep indication of who they really are, and given that the Roman Stoics believed the only true relationship we have is with ourselves, it was important that I was kind to myself and developed a decent self-opinion.

When you think about some of the comments made by your inner voice, they can be downright lacerating and fill you with self-doubt. Now, imagine for a second that this inner voice/constant critic turns its attention on a friend of yours, someone who is vulnerable. Listening to its language and seeing the effect that it is having, would you really stand by and let it carry on, or would you stand up for your friend? I'd like to think I would stand up for my friend, but about defending myself from myself I wasn't so sure. Humans are very good at finding fault with themselves, but not so good at building themselves up.

It's the relationship that you have with yourself which dictates the quality of relationships you have with other people. If you're low on self-worth, it stems from a sense of shame or regret you're carrying, which means you're allowing the past to dictate your experience of the present. You can't change what's happened, but you absolutely can change the way you experience the present. Everything we do or choose not to do radiates outwards with a ripple effect and affects other people. It's important to be able to compartmentalise, and by that I mean to be able to place any ill-feeling you might have for yourself in a box while you're dealing with it. Otherwise it can run amok and drip into other areas in which it has no place being.

When your behaviour brings into question everything who you think you are, you're in a dangerous place. Journaling helped bring me back to who I was, and reminded me of how I *usually* went about things, at least for the past fifty-four years (I'd like to think with a modicum of grace). This gave me back some confidence. Self-confidence is born from a feeling of self-worth and certitude within yourself. It allows you to recognise your strengths to try new things, to value yourself, to take time out that you might need for yourself, and to believe you are good enough and deserve to experience happiness in your life. It's amazing how journaling is able to focus on things more objectively than mere thinking, as if the distance between your brain and the pen/keyboard is sufficient for you to separate yourself at least slightly from your otherwise entirely subjective view. Self-worth is a measurer of whether we feel we are broken or working, useful or useless to others. My problem was that Parkinson's made me feel socially awkward, and uncomfortable in my skin. Because of my shakes and dyskinesia, I increasingly felt self-conscious, and uncomfortable being with people, and as a result I did the classic thing that people with Parkinson's do – I isolated myself. And when you isolate yourself, you're even more at the mercy of your low self-esteem, because it's basically saying to you, 'Here's the proof of why you are broken: you're on your own, everything's got worse and you're not worth a shit.'

Poor self-esteem is like a monkey which sits on your shoulder. It's the voice inside your head which is permanently looking for negatives and questioning everything positive that you try to come up with. MIND, the mental health organisation, suggests that sometimes we need to prove to ourselves that that monkey on our shoulder is completely wrong, and the way that we can do this is by finding evidence of other people telling us that we are worth *something*. You can look back through emails and find somebody congratulating you on a good job. Or a birthday card or a Post-it note where somebody is saying that they love you.

When I had brain surgery to help my Parkinson's in 2024, I was astounded by how many people sent me messages of heartfelt support on Instagram. I don't have much of a following on social media because I think it's unhealthy and dangerous for the mind and the soul to depend on dopamine handouts when somebody likes your picture. But what these hundred-odd comments from friends past and present did was prove to me that I meant something to other people and that I would be missed if I didn't wake up from the operation. Sometimes that's all we need to hear: that we can make a difference to others' lives. In taking away the spotlight from ourselves and putting it on others, that distracts us from our self(-ish) Self and gives us a wider sense of responsibility.

Chapter 9

Lookout Point

Time

Rumble Fish (1983), is an early Francis Ford Coppola movie and a personal favourite when nostalgia comes calling. It immediately connects me to my younger self at about nineteen or twenty. The film is peppered with close-ups of ticking clocks. It's a story about the passing of time and the brief glory of youth. Tom Waits plays 'Benny the Barman', and gives the most memorable lines of wisdom in the story: 'Time is a funny thing. Time is a very peculiar item. You see, when you're young, you're a kid, you've got time, you got nothing but time. Throw away a couple of years here, a couple of years there. It doesn't matter. [But] the older you get you say, "Jesus, how much I got? I got thirty-five summers left." Thirty-five summers ... Think about it!'

I was thinking about it, time was catching up with me and I didn't have thirty-five summers left. Unlike before the diagnosis with Parky, when I was profligate with my health and time, forever considering myself a durable specimen of the human race, I was now under no such illusions. I was much more aware of what was passing than ever before, and also what I was losing. Time nipped ferally at my heels, reminding me with regularity that my lifespan was going to be shorter than the average person's because of this condition which had developed seemingly from out of the blue.

The lifespan of an average person with Parkinson's Disease is twenty years. You end up developing pneumonia after a fall or an illness and then you die, or you swallow your food the wrong way and it ends up entering a lung. I'm not looking into it. Why would I want to research my end? Instead, I have kept telling myself that I'm not the *average* person, and that I have pushed the envelope so much further than the average person on so many occasions over the last decade or more of having this damned disease. Now, whenever I started taking time for granted and days were wasted in depression, self-pity and resentment, I began instead to embrace the thought of my probable expiry date as a kind of wake-up gift. Just like the last couple of After Eights in that dark interior of the box are always the best tasting because you know they will all soon be gone.

Perhaps it was because both my son's and my own birthday were drawing close that I was thinking about time on this particular trip up to Skye, but I could hear the sand shifting ever south in an hourglass in the back of my mind; one marked with my name on it.

The Roman Stoic Seneca once said that the problem with humans, 'is not that we have a short space of time, but that we waste so much of it.'

I wonder why we always think we need more, and why we are unsatisfied with what we have. In my case, the displeasure was all about time; or the lack of time I had allotted for my son Finn and I to get to Skye and back again. We were going there for just two days' swimming and walking, with a day's travel each side. The problem wasn't the time, it was more how much we were attempting to squeeze into that period. And that is not, or should not, be what wild swimming is about, at least in my book. For in nature, when you give it a chance, time is like the hands of the clock being dipped in honey, weighing it down and slowing the incessant urgency.

Nature has this brilliant way of bringing you back to a slower walking pace than you find yourself usually moving at; the speed of life. Trying to cram too much in is almost as bad as wasting time; either way you're not making the most of whatever it is that you're doing, nor are you taking things at the right speed to enjoy yourself. And all the stress and fatigue that followed our trip was because I hadn't given us much time. The fact that we had loads of time months before, when we had plenty of windows in which we could have gone to Skye was immaterial. True, I had been waiting for confirmation on my deep brain surgery, which was moved from November to early December, then on to my birthday (10 January), and then again into February. So, to cut Finn and I a little bit of slack, things had been somewhat up in the air, and my health seemed to have got worse over the last six months after separating with M.

There are certain people who flourish creatively at the eleventh hour. It's not because they are lazy or chancers, it's because when they're under pressure they seem to produce their best work. I am like this with my magazine and newspaper articles; it's as if I leave the stories to germinate in my mind for as long as possible, and then at the last minute a green shoot of an idea appears and then grows very quickly into a full-bodied article in just two drafts. This doesn't condone being late for a flight. I simply seem to be more comfortable being last-minute-Jack. Why?

Finn and I were late getting to Bristol Airport because we'd been arsing about trying to pick up a drone camera that had been purchased online from Curry's but hadn't yet arrived at the house in Cirencester. We needed it because Finn was to shoot a short film to accompany this book. We had to take a diversion to another store that cost us valuable time and meant we arrived dangerously close to the allotted check-in time. In fact, the check-in had already closed.

'What is it about you, me and planes, son?' Were we in this position because we'd stopped to get the drone and the staff took forever to fetch it, or was it perhaps something a little more serious? Finn, like his father, shares a trait not altogether helpful in these modern times of digital precision; he has no idea of time. That's a nice way of saying he's always late. As am I, though less often these days and to explain I hope you'll indulge me telling you a wee story.

The first book I ever ghost-wrote was a modest little tome called *Stand Up Straight*. It was intended to be a sibling read to complement the brilliant *Make Your Bed* written by ex-Navy Seal William H. McRaven, which had become an international bestseller. His book focused on the transferable values of the elite Navy Seals which could be used in civilian life. Mine would be very much the same, though instead of Navy Seals, it would draw its wisdom from the Royal Military Academy Sandhurst.

I was to meet the academy's commandant, Major General Paul Nanson, at midday sharp. The editor I was working with arranged to meet me there, and as I drove up to the Gurkhas on vigil at the gate, I was early. But then I went to Old College building instead of New College, or was it the other way around? The problem was 'new college' looked more like an old college and I was now suddenly out of comfy time and late, but had to drive at a crawl to the other side of the spacious campus, observing the 20 mph speed limit. Next, I had to find the room we were meeting in.

I was now five minutes late, and as I knocked on a thick oak door a voice from beyond, deep as a Shakespearean actor's, boomed at me to enter. There, in a wood-panelled room dominated by a table longer than a longship, sat the major general wearing an expression like a torn sheet, accompanied by his aide, who was equally unimpressed by my tardiness. Opposite them sat my editor. I had failed my first test at Sandhurst. Still, at least I managed to get there in the end, even if it had taken me thirty years to do so!

After a brief chat about the book, we were to write together if – and it was still a big *if*, I was approved – polite chat revealed that we had played rugby against one another's schools, both of which were in Lancashire. He visibly softened, and then asked me if I would like to have a driven tour of the campus, stopping off at the key places like the New College and the parade ground where officers passed out before joining their chosen regiment. An hour later, having been driven by a dangerous-looking valet/bodyguard with an exaggerated boxer's nose, the commandant had taken the measure of me and obviously reflected that there was more to this guy with a shaking hand than just being late for meetings. He was an impressive character, clearly very popular with his staff and beyond the mask and facade of authority, he seemed like a really decent bloke.

The tour now finished, we returned to the publisher in the wood-panelled room, clearly inquisitive as to whether the big cheese of Sandhurst and I had got on or not. Major General Nanson *had* clicked well enough with me for him to report we would make a good team. A palpable wave of relief followed from my editor, and with a handshake and a gentlemen's agreement we left. Over the next few months, in email exchanges and a couple of return visits to the campus, overnighting at the commandant's house, we explored the different values that were instilled in the rough lads who were eventually shaped into officers. One of those values was time. Being late and making someone wait for you, said Major General Nanson, was akin to stealing that person's time, because while they're waiting for you they are effectively held captive, unable to do anything else or go anywhere else, all because of your lack of discipline. As an effective aid against being late and letting others down, at the academy they preach something called 'Sandhurst Time', which essentially means arriving 10 minutes earlier than your allotted appointment. This gives you time to compose, straighten up, be your relaxed self and not start off on a bad foot. And it applies to everything in your life, from arriving at a train station to meeting a friend, or even turning up for a battle. By making this 10-minute breather into a habit, you respect other people's time and yourself. Since learning of this, I've been late many times but considerably less, now that I think of myself as a thief not just of my time, but other people's, too.

The plane from Bristol Airport almost didn't land at Inverness, our staging post for the Hebrides archipelago, because of poor visibility. The pilot was talking about switching our route to Edinburgh and a collective groan swept through the small plane. This particular trip to the

Isle of Skye was going to be a whistle-stop visit and only afforded us two days' swimming. So to lose just one day would be catastrophic, not to mention being a very expensive exercise for such a short period. Time was precious and couldn't be wasted on buses from Edinburgh to Inverness the next day; we had to be in Skye tonight. *Ah shit!* Those words of Mike Tyson's which I'd quoted myriad times while writing other people's books came back to me as though writ in neon: 'Everyone has a plan until they get punched in the mouth.'

A plan is just that, it's nothing certain. And when you put yourself in a position which allows for nothing to go wrong, that's when you start to constrict with inner tension and begin displaying signs of external stress; you become inflexible and combustible, like a car's water tank overheating. So I did what I always do in situations where the outcome is entirely out of my hands; I handed it over to the universe, and said to myself, 'Whatever happens I'll make the best of it. It may not be what was planned, and it might be a pain in the neck, but there will be a lesson in here somewhere for me. It's already written and decided if we're to make it to Skye tonight.'

Luckily, this evening father and son were favoured by Hermes and successfully arrived at their chosen and now mist-free rendezvous with the Viking, whom we spotted by the baggage reclaim, hidden under a trucker's cap. Inverness Airport had become so familiar on my many trips to the Isle of Skye over the last couple of years. Finn and Matt had met for the first time earlier in the year during summer and they gave each other a massive bear hug. By now, after a number of trips, I not only trusted his detailed knowledge of Skye with my son's safety and mine, but I could also number Matt among the few people I can genuinely call friends.

He had already driven an hour to get here without complaint, and would now have a further two-and-a-half hours' drive through the highlands and on to Skye itself, then all the way up to its northerly point, which looks out upon the neighbouring Isles of Lewis and Harris. Also joining us on this trip was Matt's son Fergus, a polite and gentle giant with dreadlocks. Diagnosed with ADHD, he was animated by his passion for music, and not afraid to ask any question, given that lens through which he saw life had an altogether different filter than a non-neurodiverse person. From the instant Finn and I met him, his honesty was a breath of fresh air; his relentless curiosity didn't stop until he was at the nub of a thing, and his thoroughness had a way of making you re-examine certain things you might have taken for granted. Wherever Fergus went, so did his sound bath drum. Finn had taught himself to play the guitar during the COVID-19 pandemic, and like Fergus seemed to possess a natural aptitude for music. The two young men chatted about chords, keys and bands in the back of Matt's jeep as he drove through the dark winter night towards the fabled island.

'I may not be a very good wingman tonight,' I said. 'Sorry, but I'm knackered, pal. Haven't been sleeping much lately.'

'I've got something that will help you sleep.' Matt grinned like a demented badger, the car's dial lights pooling green in his glasses, 'We'll have a doobie before we crash later,' he said conspiratorially.

I noticed his hand tremoring. 'How are your shakes pal?' I asked.

The grin fell away, 'They've been getting a bit worse. When I was in Mexico City recently to drum up some inspiration for my sculpture, they sort of took over one day and I had to call my wife Michelle who was with the kids in Scotland. The reason for the shakes being that bad, I mean my whole body was shaking terribly, was because I can't sleep without a bit of weed to send me off, and I'd been in Mexico City for about a week.'

I swooned, 'A week in Mexico City, at that altitude without sleep? You must have been exhausted!'

He nodded, 'Yeah, I was, and as you warned me, it makes sense to be mindful of where you walk and who's around you.'

Matt is the kind of bloke who when he smiles it's hard not to be warmed by it. If he accidentally found himself stepping through a bad neighbourhood, of which Mexico City has a fair few, he did so with the right mix of curiosity, friendliness and surety of direction to get out of it.

'Yes,' I agreed, 'you have to pretend you have a sense of purpose. Even if you don't.'

Matt nodded and said, 'There are more art museums per square foot in Mexico City than any other city on earth. I was walking from one to the other every day, sometimes for miles and miles. Looking around you, being constantly vigilant, is mentally tiring, especially with no sleep, and one day my body had finally had enough and said, "Right, that's it, I'm not moving any further until I get some proper rest."'

'So what did you do?' I asked.

'Well, it finally occurred to me that cannabis isn't actually banned in Mexico; it's legal to buy it at the counter, so I went and got some, rolled an epic doobie and slept like a baby that night.'

'And the shakes?' I asked.

'They behaved themselves.' He smiled.

'How are the shakes at the moment?' I asked.

'Okay,' he said, 'I've been told I am pre-Diabetes so it's connected with that. It's up to me to follow the advice and get myself right.'

We stared at the open moorland ahead of us, desolate and black. I yawned massively.

'Look, you best try and catch some kip on the way, pal, as once we get to the northern tip of Skye we've a walk to get to the bothy.'

'A long walk?'

'Well, I'm not going to lie to you, it's not short,' he answered.

I groaned.

'Trust me, it will be worth it just for the view in the morning,' he added.

As the road cut and snaked through an impossibly dense forest on each side of the car, we passed signposts to places straight from the pages of Macbeth, one of which was Cawdor, and then another, Glamis. *Ear of newt, wing of bat,* I thought to myself.

I closed my eyes to try and still my tremor so I could sleep. No sooner had I done so than the boys in the back erupted with excitement. Apparently, a red stag had appeared from the impenetrable black wall of forest at roadside, huge and stately, his horns wide and regal.

'Seven pointer that,' said Matt.

'What's a seven pointer?' asked Fergus.

'It means it's got seven sharp points on each side of its antlers.'

'Do they get more points as they become older?'

'No, age has got nothing to do with it,' said Matt. 'Believe it or not, the red deer loses his horns every year and regrows them. The velvet stage is when they first grow and they're smooth as silk to the touch.'

'Wouldn't that be dangerous?' asked Fergus.

'Sorry, I'm being a bit literal,' Matt corrected himself. 'But you wouldn't want to get so close to a male that you could touch his horns.'

Fergus poked his head above the stack of bags he and Finn were sharing the backseat with. 'Literal and figurative have now become interchangeable … since 1913. I think that's right, I'll have to come back to you on that, so don't quote me.'

'I won't,' said Matt. 'Anyway, compared to the velvet stage, when a stag sheds his antlers after the rutting season, they end up a fleshy, oozy pulp.'

I closed my eyes again, and a mile or so further on yet another set of white-green eyes were caught in the headlights. I'd missed the nocturnal treat again. 'Maybe it was a wendigo?' I mumbled.

'Nah,' said Finn, 'you only get wendigo in the States and Canada.'

'I didn't mean it literally,' I yawned.

We rolled on.

My hand was shaking more this time than on the previous visit during summer; every time I came here, like a child's increasing height measurements recorded on a kitchen wall, the island charted my gradual decline. And just as my understanding and attachment to the island deepened, so did the tentacles of my illness spread. On my right arm was a tattoo of a sperm whale. It had been inspired by a scrimshaw I'd seen in Martha's Vineyard. Scrimshaws were the yellow teeth of dead sperm whales that harpooners engraved with ships and creatures of the deep, whiling away the hours in the doldrums if there was no wind. In the days of whaling, sperm whales, those colossal regents of the deep, were harpooned and slaughtered in their millions for their spermaceti oil which was used for candle wax; at one time the world's illumination depended on it.

In 2014, I'd been on one of my favourite assignments for the *Daily Telegraph*, to Martha's Vineyard island,

Cape Cod. I was on the boat of a wonderful couple called Lisa and Buddy Vanderhoop. We were talking Great Whites and looking at the remains of the *Orca*, the ill-fated boat in *Jaws*, which was rotting on the opposite bank of the estuary that runs past Menemsha dock. Like in Hemingway's *The Old Man and the Sea*, where a magnificent marlin is tied to Santiago's little boat but is filched by sharks, there was very little of the original sailing craft left thanks to cinephiles who sneaked off with bits of the boat as keepsakes. Buddy's mooring point was exactly where Quint's workshop was in the film. Buddy is a Wampanoag Native American whose great uncle Amos Smalley, a skilled harpooner, had a story uncannily close to that of Tashtego, one of Herman Melville's characters in *Moby Dick*. According to Buddy, he had killed a real white whale just off the Azores, and to prove it, the charismatic captain – who was one of the survivors caught out at sea in the 1991 *Perfect Storm* – reached in his pocket and withdrew a huge yellow tooth ornamented with a scrimshaw.

The tattoo at the top of my right arm portrays a sperm whale locked in fierce battle with a giant squid, its tentacles wrapped tight around the cetacean. It's hard to tell who's winning; some days the whale looks as if it has the edge, while on others the squid seems to be throttling the whale, much like my good days and bad days with PD. My reason for getting inked was that I needed a daily reminder that this disease could be fought, even though, like the tentacles of the squid, it would come at me from all angles. It was a battle for the long haul.

As far as long hauls went, Matt seemed to have spirited us supernaturally quickly to the Kyle of Lochalsh. The word comes from the Gaelic *caol*, meaning narrow strait. The Isle of Skye is extremely close to the mainland and as soon as the car sped up the smooth arch of Skye Bridge it felt regenerative. Skye holds a charge of energy unlike any other place and as the jeep touched down upon the ageless granite of the island, on cue I fell fast asleep.

Time teaches us life's most important lessons, but it's only with the luxury of hindsight that we can look back on events and understand why things happened just the way they did. At the time it can feel difficult, unfair and painful, but this is part of the scheme of things. When you start to piece together these landmarks in your life, which at the time may have appeared completely isolated and random, and you can join up the dots, then you begin to see the magic of the universe; *nothing* happens by accident. And time creates constellations at her own pace, she cannot be hurried.

I couldn't remember how many times I'd been to Skye, just that each time it seemed to be with a different hat on; first, as a travel journalist, then an author ghostwriting an ex-special forces soldier's life (which surprisingly was to become a bestselling book); then, as a father trying to mend his broken relationship with his son; next as an author researching this book. But whatever the hat and my reason for being here, I was always a supplicant of the regenerative powers of this wild and dramatic island.

I seem to remember Matt saying, 'We're here,' feeling as if I had only just manged to get some sleep, and then looking at the glowing clock which now read 2 a.m. Standing in the corner of the car park at the northernmost point of the Isle of Skye, and like a solitary Coldstream Guard resplendent in red livery, stood a lonely telephone box. It was the last bastion of civilisation that we'd see for the next hour as we tramped through bogs. We were on the much fabled Trotternish Peninsula, home to a landscape of rock pinnacles, barrow-like mounds and basalt cliffs, the most northerly point of which is Rubha Hunish.

In the darkness, pitch-black but for our little torches, we unloaded our essential kit from the bags we'd brought with us from England into the more portable rucksacks which contained a sleeping bag and a floor mat Matt had already packed for us.

'How far did you say it was, mate?' I asked Matt.

'I reckon we can do it in an hour and a half, but let's see how we get on,' he answered.

'Do you think it will be busy?' I enquired.

'I'd be very surprised if there's anyone there; hopefully we'll have the place to ourselves.'

Finn was quiet. I had a feeling he was coming down with something; I'd been dosing him up with cold and 'flu remedy, coupled with healthy smoothie drinks, in an attempt to stave off the arrival of aching joints.

'Okay son?' I asked.

'I'm fine,' he replied grimly, and I didn't believe a word of it.

Off we tramped like a caravan of fireflies, the muddy peat making sucking sounds as it hungrily swallowed our boots. I was deliriously tired; I didn't have the energy to walk or climb uphill for an hour. As Matt and Fergus disappeared into the night, Finn waited patiently for me. I was out of puff and wobbly, but worst of all was my dyskinesia which was making me very wobbly and throwing my balance off guard. The pack I was carrying wasn't especially heavy, but there were rocks and puddles and bogs to jump across. The blessing that comes with walking in the darkness is you can't see how far you've got to left to walk.

Remember Rich, I told myself dramatically, *this place is where your ancestors are from, this is the wellspring and it can make you feel better and stronger than any other place.* And with that, I slipped on a rock and flew backwards as I lost my footing. Breathless, I sat down to gather any strength I had left. God, I hated this disease that made me so tired. I felt like screaming. The ascent was brutal at times, my legs rubbery and weak I as teetered, about to fall backwards. Each time my son was behind me to catch my back and push me forward. 'Come on Dad, we're nearly there,' he encouraged.

Ahead of us, I sensed the sea. It was so utterly black we could have been inches from the edge of a cliff and not known it. At the top of the next rise the squat form of the bothy appeared with the slyness of a ghost ship. Finn put his arm around my shoulder. 'We made it!'

I sighed with relief and the knowledge that I had nothing left in the tank – my body was now running on fumes. I was last into the bothy, but soon had to back up as the former coastguard building was full to the gills with bodies in sleeping bags. Every spot taken, the wet and freezing floor was our only option. It was now the middle of the night. Matt volunteered to return to the car and sleep there while Finn and Fergus and I unrolled our floor mats and tried to blow them up as quietly as possible. It was so cold in there we could see our breath in the torchlight. Sleep did not come easily. I spent most of the remaining hours wriggling around in my sleeping bag trying to get comfortable, too tired to allow myself to sleep.

It didn't help that at about 8 a.m. the pupae started to hatch from their sleeping bags and woke us up. A hand was tapping me insistently on the shoulder and asking me to move so they could get out of the door. Groggy, I opened my eyes to a grey dawn. My eye sockets felt as if they had been scooped out. The prospect of getting into cold water could not have been more unappealing. After the mass exodus from the bothy, we had a little more sleep and then I managed to unpeel myself from my sleeping bag and get dressed. It was tiny in there. From the outside, the building more resembled a boat, 'It reminds me of the *Orca* in *Jaws*,' said Matt, who had returned to the bothy. And then I started singing 'Fare well and adieu to you fair Spanish ladies, farewell and adieu to you ladies of Spain ...'

From the bothy there was the most extraordinary view of the cliffs far below and of the islands of Harris and Lewis just opposite. From here, on a lucky day, you can see migrating orca, humpback whales, porpoise and dolphin and, as was the case today, the spectral form of surfacing submarines. Two popped up to say hello while I was getting changed. Of course, I never saw them; the early bird gets the worm, and it was Matt who espied them, so close, he said, that he could almost read the white paint lettering on their coal-black hides.

We sat in the lookout room drinking up the wide-screen views afforded by windows on three sides. A real 180 degree viewpoint, this bothy is considered to be the most scenic in the whole of Scotland. Upon one wall there's a wonderful illustrated poster of the cetacean family with the whales' true size shown relative to each other, so you can accurately compare each species. I'd seen humpback whales, or rather heard them through the fog when I was in Provincetown, Cape Cod. It wasn't until thirty years later that I was lucky enough to see them fairly up close in Iceland. And then there were the sperm whales with whom I'd been privileged to free dive in the Caribbean; the highlight of which was being 30 feet down close beside a mother and her calf. The patient way she studied me with her all-seeing grey eye was like connecting with the mystery of the universe. To think that out of this bothy's windows you can spot so many passing giants is unfathomable. There were so many other whales I wanted to see before my last sunset.

Mid-morning, we made to leave Rubha Hunish, but not before a swim to give us some much needed zest. The wind was up as we made for the ashen-black ruins of Duntulm Castle. Originally an Iron Age *broch* (fortified house), it was later used by the Norsemen, but what little remains today are the fifteenth-century tower and seventeenth-century walls framing the courtyard. Built on a basalt promontory, its black ruined walls are part of the mythic fabric which makes this island so special.

It looks like the crib of the Kurgan, the villain to Connor MacLeod's hero in the film *Highlander* (1986). If you want to find that, you'll have to head to Castle Tioram in Loch Moidart in the Highlands. As to Connor MacLeod's beautiful castle where he gets married in the film, that sits opposite the bridge to Skye in the Kyle of Lochalsh and is called Eilean Donan Castle.

Duntulm Castle is said to be one of the most haunted places in Scotland, but if I had a fiver for every time I heard that I'd never have to work again. Resident ghosts include a ham-fisted nurserymaid who somehow dropped a baby out of the ramparts and was murdered in reprisal. It's said her screams haunt the castle on a stormy night. That said, they have to compete with the groans of an imprisoned MacDonald who was fed salt beef and no water, and the ghosts of a man named Donald Form and his revelling companions down in the wine cellar. Oh, and a wandering one-eyed woman.

Duntulm ruins sit on a promontory, and given that a chunk of it last fell on to the rocks below as late as 1990, it is best to heed the warning signs and not step foot on it. It's a bit of a wander down the cliff to the beach. The water was moss-green in the changing light of the sky. Reluctantly, I slid into the shallows. The sea's bony fingers gripped my body in a freezing embrace and got straight to work, quickening my heartbeat and stealing my breath. I checked both, forcing myself to relax by controlling my breath. I slowly counted my way through thirty 'Mississippis', suffering the initial period of discomfort, knowing that I would have to stick with it till I got to the other side. And then I dipped the final third of me up to my neck. By the time I reached the count of 'thirty Mississippi', the panic had retracted its hold and the delicious tingle of blood capillaries rushing to my extremities had started to set in. It was like drinking a huge bottle of Lucozade. I seemed to have banished my sleepiness by being in the sea and my body felt awake once more. Pure soul tonic! Finn decided against going in, preferring to check he had all the filming kit, but he still made a point of sticking his head in a rock pool of cold water to wake up. Just doing this still activates the vagus nerve which manages communications from our gut and also the fight/flight reflex. The more that we use it, the more familiar it gets with dealing with stress, and ultimately we can finesse our gut's reaction to stress in a way that we are more able to deal with real stress when it arrives, because it's now less of a stranger.

On the rocky shore south of the ruins are some remnants of Skye's former residents from the Jurassic Age. Dinosaurs, including sauropods and theropods, walked the Isle of Skye 170 million years ago, and their footprints, which are still there, can be seen at low tide if you wander out a bit.

Like looking at stars and trying to compute the mere idea that the universe might be infinite, time is something I have a mental block with when I try to imagine any span much beyond one thousand years. In the comparatively short space of the past fourteen years, Parkinson's had tried to destroy my brain, the energy and strength in my body and, at times, my will to live; variously using its wide arsenal of tricks. In that brief period, I had also allowed it to break up my family. Fortunately, I'm a great believer in finding the good within the bad, and what the last dozen years had taught me was that I was determined to ensure that the rest of my time on this planet was well spent.

Chapter 10

Camasunary Bay

Digging Deep

We all have a lot more fuel in our tanks than we realise. We are rarely forced into a survival situation where we have to dig so deep that we realise that our reservoirs of mental strength and physical stamina are far beyond that which we thought we possessed. Like a modern car when the amber light pops on warning you that you're almost empty of fuel, the manufacturer has a contingency built in; there's more left in there than the needle suggests. We, too, are capable of doing things we never thought possible. Someone once said, 'On the other side of extreme difficulty lies greatness.' It's only by going to this place of extreme hardship that we get a glimpse of who we really are, and what we can be.

Hardship, in whatever shape or form, can be good for us. If it's a lack of money you're experiencing, you soon realise you don't need half the stuff that you buy when there's plenty of money in your account. Hunger, too, can be good, in so far as it creates an appetite by which you enjoy your food more and with greater appreciation when you eventually get to eat.

From Duntulm Castle, after a brief kip and filming session, we made the half-hour trip to Portree to stock up on supplies. Then we drove to our next target, the car park on the road from Broadford to Elgol, where we would park the jeep overnight and leave it, as we made the 9-kilometre long walk to Camasunary Beach. This secluded cove sits on the Strathaird peninsula as you head south, and is reached by walking among the forbidding Cuillin mountains to the north of it.

The walk at night can seem twice as long. The pass, known as Am Mam, takes you through breathtaking views of the sea and copper-and-black peaks of the Cuillin. It's so definitively picturesque that you feel like you've walked into an old postcard. On a good day it should take about two-and-a-half hours without stopping. However, it was almost dark when we set out for the bothy by Camasunary Bay, and the landscape was a mush of wet bogs and over-flowing streams caused by unremitting rainfall. The night was bleak with barely a star to light our way.

Not far from here, on the other side of the mountain, was creepy Loch Coruisk. Tonight, with the sky black as tar, we could see very little in front of us, bar our torch-light and the steam coming from our breath as we humped heavy packs up the steep, slippery path which wound its way up the mountain. I was in a foul mood, purely because I was exhausted. Finny was quiet, as were Fergus and Matt.

None of us had slept well the night before in the Lookout Bothy, and so it was all we could do now just to keep one leg moving in front of the other. It had been a much later departure time than we had intended, but light being so short-lived in the Hebrides come February, and with filming having to be completed at the Lookout Bothy, our lack of sleep had impacted heavily on us. Everything we did was now at half speed.

Within 10 minutes' walk from the car park on the road from Broadford to Elgol, we came to a stream that had overflown its banks. For some reason, Finn had bought trainers with him, rather than a sturdy pair of waterproof boots, and in no time his feet were soaking. A few minutes later, so was the rest of him as the rain continued to fall loudly all around us. The path we followed lurched up and down like a rollercoaster track and we were stopping every 100 yards, our calf muscles screaming, our backs groaning with the weight of our backpacks. Finn insisted on carrying the filming kit in addition to his rucksack and each time I offered to take it for a while, he refused.

I literally had nothing left in the tank and that made me resentful and bad tempered as we slipped and fell in the dark. Back in the old days before this damn disease I could've kept going – my reserves were much deeper then – and I had tramped through more steaming jungles than I cared to remember. And yet now, PD had me by the short and curlies: my fatigue levels were off the scale, I was the weakest member of the group and it felt as if I was breathing with only one lung. To make matters worse, my whole body was possessed by dyskinesia, which kept making me feel I was about to fall backwards. I would try to balance myself with my arms like some sea bird caught in a foul wind, struggling desperately to right itself with its wings. I felt puppeteer-ed by the dyskinesia, the way it created a spectacle of flailing limbs, which I was always trying to control. The symptoms were getting worse, and stress adding to this and exacerbating them.

Sometimes you can find yourself in a situation that is so appalling, you can almost taste the future and nostalgia in it; then you either laugh or cry because it's so bloody ridiculous or unpleasant. I knew that night that I was scraping the barrel in terms of the energy that I had available, and there were times I found myself sitting on a wet tussock of grass at the side of the path like a gladiator having a time-out before going back into the madness of the fight. We began to spread out, each of us locked in his own personal challenge against the wet night and the climb. And then Fergus's rucksack strap broke and shortly after, not far from the apex of the path, his torch lost power and he fell over. The night was so pitch black that to the left side of the path was just a shapeless abyss.

I was reminded of the Stoic philosopher Epictetus's advice that in adversity you find you have strengths you never realised. However inelegant I was in my ascent, and however much poisonous invective flew out of my mouth as I cursed the mountain, wind and rain, one thing that this beast of a walk was teaching me was that despite this illness I now had, the mountain had not yet broken me, and I was still in possession of the guts that I'd always had. I was being forced to recalibrate my expectations of what I was capable of. It seemed like on the basis of tonight, I had been underestimating myself. I would get there in the end, even if that meant suffering considerably more punish-ment than my body could afford; I would not be beaten by myself. This wasn't just an exhausting and, some might say, long foolhardy trek by night; it was a war cry to my fading body that my spirit was still strong, and I was not the shuffling ape I sometimes saw myself as.

When we finally made it to the top, Matt's torch had also lost power and shortly after, so too did mine. The path disappeared into the future; we could literally see it, swal-lowed by the darkness. Finn and I shared his torch and carried the film kit bag between us. Now the challenge was not to slip on the lethal downward track, which ran slick with rainwater and with jagged stones poking out at every angle like collapsing headstones. However perilous the gradient was, in another hour we had completed our descent and were at the root of the mountain on the flat, but for the moment we had lost Matt and Fergus. Finn and I found ourselves walking up and down small hillocks, wandering towards a distant light. It was the wrong light and not that of the bothy, but rather a small farm, whose owner was responsible for creating the path we had just scaled, for his Land Rover. It was hard to imagine somebody having the balls to drive even a Land Rover down such extreme gradients and I take my hat off to those extraordinary machines – now sadly no longer in production – for being such capable workhorses.

Whether it was Finn or me, I can't remember, but one of us finally managed to persuade the other that we were walking towards the sea, and would soon be in it. Mist was closing in around us, a thickening sea fog tumbling over the tops of the nearby waves, but at least it had now stopped raining. From a distance, we heard Matt calling out to us, while Finn's torch-light fell upon what looked like an emaciated and very inebriated Father Christmas passed out in a face plant on the moor. It turned out to be a squashed street cone and some flotsam that had gathered on the corner of the beach. Amazing what the imagination can conjure up.

Having rediscovered the correct path, which made a sharp left turn we had failed to follow, we were now able to see another light, and this time it was the right one; that of the bothy. It's hard to describe the sense of relief that I experienced when I realised the trial was finally over. As the bothy grew in definition the closer we got to it, so too did our sense of jubilation. Halfway towards the light we were met by the Viking, who had been looking for us. 'Bloody hell lads, you had me worried,' he said breathlessly. 'I changed the batteries of the torch and was combing the beach for you.'

Finn looked over at me, I think he winked. 'Funny you should say that.'

Once inside the bothy, we were almost too tired to speak and barely managed to say 'hello' to a gathering of young people on a school reunion.

After our experience sleeping on the floor at Lookout Point, there were more important things to do than make conversation with the other inhabitants, and that meant finding a berth for the night before any other travellers turned up out of the darkness. While Matt decided on setting out his bed in the little ante-room by the front door, where everybody left their boots, Fergus, Finn and I had the top deck of the bunks to ourselves, basically a wooden platform that could comfortably have slept six.

Candles flickered, creating shadows on the walls of the bothy as a fresh assault of rain pelted the windows. That's the problem with bothies, the lack of electric light. So, when there are lots of people crammed into one, it's very easy to end up putting your stuff in someone else's rucksack, because lined up against the dormitory walls in low light, they all tend to look the same. The night in the Lookout Bothy, an exhausted Finn had taken off his rings and carefully put them inside what he thought was the front pocket of his rucksack, but which sadly turned out to belong to someone else who had long left the building by the time Finn realised his mistake next morning, Tonight, I was so tired after the punishing odyssey in the mountains, that I found myself pulling out someone else's fresh underpants and socks from what I thought was my bag.

When I finally located the correct rucksack in the half-light, I also quickly realised that while sorting my bag earlier on in the car park before we set off, I must have taken out and forgotten to repack my washbag, which contained not only my emergency supply of day meds, but the night meds, whose purpose was to keep me still at night so I might catch some sleep. By this stage of the illness, each day I was taking about twenty pills, made up of seven different types: a mix of meds in the morning to get me started, some more to give me energy, others to give me replacement feel-good vibes because my body no longer produced dopamine, some to keep me still, yet others to keep me going. It was this cocktail of different meds that caused the side effect of dyskinesia; ironically one of the worst symptoms.

Although I was exhausted, I still had enough energy left in me to panic. And I was panicking now because tonight was a perfect opportunity to recharge my batteries, but by leaving that bloody washbag in the car, I had now consigned myself to eight hours of shaking, with three swims intended for tomorrow and then the 9.2-kilometre slog back across those effing mountains. I would be dead. Sleep is such a difficult commodity to get when you have Parkinson's. In pursuit of it in the past I took some lamentable risks which could have gone horribly wrong. At one point, the only way I found I could really get some zeds was by taking a tincture of cannabis oil with the THC left in it (THC is the bit which can get you stoned). The sooner they change the legislation so people with severe conditions can be licensed to carry it on long-haul journeys, and to their forward destinations, the better for everyone; especially those on the flight who sit in front, behind and next to you! The problem was knowing how much of it to use because it's very strong stuff. Consequently, I had a few mishaps along the way, like when I had to go and do a training job in a well-known psychiatric hospital (for the criminally insane). The place was so creepy it could screw with your head even without taking cannabis. It was an early start, still dark, I was driving towards the motorway and realised I was *accidentally* stoned. I put all the car's windows down to wake me up. I was now on the M4 and spears of magnesium white light were burning towards me, as if I was flying at warp speed at the controls of the Millennium Falcon. I quickly checked the speed dial – I was doing 20 mph, puttering along like a granny in the slow lane as cars and lorries thundered past me!

Another time I was travelling for work through Sydney Airport when I had to walk directly past the head of a sniffer dog which was checking everybody as they passed through a tight exit. Its owner was brandishing a machine gun. I had some of the cannabis oil in my hand luggage, only a couple of dots as tiny as spots on a domino – in this case on a few bourbon biscuits wrapped in foil – but it was cannabis oil all the same. The dog must have had a cold; it let me go.

One good thing that I did do during this fourteen-year journey was getting myself on a drug trial which used a medication already on the market. It was really empowering to know I was doing my bit to combat the disease, and not just sitting back and letting it infect and weaken me. The drug being trialled was called Exenatide and usually used for people suffering from Type 2 Diabetes. The medication was a cloned version of the spit of a Gila monster. Allegedly, Gila monsters, ugly black and yellow lizards which live in the Mexican deserts, eat only two or three times a year and are particularly adept at controlling their sugar levels. By chance, doctors prescribing Exenatide to people with Type 2 Diabetes who also happened to have Parkinson's, noticed that the drug had seemingly improved their patients' tremor and motor skills. Because the drug has already been through the endlessly slow palaver of being tested and released on the market, it could soon be a game changer.

I was told I had got on the Exenatide trial and that it would last eighteen months. It was 2015, and I was silly busy with work. In that year alone I worked in Crete, Ionian Greece, Paris, New York, Boston, Laos, Borneo and Zurich. I asked if it was okay for me to take it abroad on assignments, and the doctors organising the trial were fine with that. The Exenatide trial was known as a *double placebo*, which meant that even the neurologists officiating the trial in Queen Square didn't know who was taking the placebo and who was taking the genuine drug, as it arrived pre-packaged from the US. If you were really unlucky, you could go the whole eighteen months injecting yourself in the stomach every day with nothing but saline. Any recovery was down to you and the powers of self-kidology – aka placebo – rather than the drugs.

The trial was conducted in the new wing of Queen Square, in a ward known as the Wolfstone Clinic. It was a welcoming place I looked forward to going to, and the staff were good people. I loved being fussed over and it was very high tech; with the mere touch of a button they could frost the windows up for immediate privacy.

During the eighteen-month period of the trial, I stopped drinking coffee because the smell alone made me nauseous (a side-effect of Exenatide), and I was regularly sick and vomiting (also side-effects of the drug). But on a positive note, I experienced a real flush of increased energy, so that even when I went to Sabah in Borneo for Lonely Planet, I was marching through equatorial jungles like a teenager. And between occasionally having my head down the hotel toilet vomiting while I learnt my PADI open water theory, my virgin scuba was at Sipadan Island once described by Jacques Cousteau as 'an untouched piece of art', where I got to glide over a technicolour reef swarming with black-tip and reef sharks, octopus and cuttlefish. Curiously, on the surface of tiny Sipadan Island, there were armed soldiers with guns trained on the watery horizon to stop Filipino pirates from kidnapping unexpecting surfacing divers.

I also noticed how much I had changed in my attitude towards strangers living with a disability. Where before there would have been pity if I noticed them at all, now there was empathy. I remember a man in his twenties burning up in the intense sun, balanced on crutches. It was in a place called Kota Kinabalu, Sabah's capital city, and he was selling pens. I walked by, and as he offered me a cheap biro he accidentally dropped a box of them on the ground. They scattered everywhere. I asked him to relax while I quickly picked them all up. Then I bought ten of them. I imagined my Aggie standing there in his place, forced to do the same.

On my eventual return to the Wolfstone Clinic, I was subjected to lots of tests before finally stopping taking the medicine. It was eventually revealed to me that my motor skills had improved by 19 per cent, but that I had been on a placebo all along. That was an extraordinary feat of change – 19 per cent recovery had only happened by my being completely clear in my mind that I was on the real thing. After I knew I wasn't on Exenatide, I was no longer actively fooling myself that I was getting better, so naturally I began to lose what I had gained from self-healing.

It wasn't just the placebo which was able to give me hope, I took it where I could find it and from the strangest of sources. In the spring of 2016, I was working in Denver and had a few days' holiday after finishing so I could do a commission for *iNews* on the renowned and downright creepy Stanley Hotel. Forced to turn back by an oncoming snowstorm, Stephen King had stayed one night here with his wife and young son. A skeleton staff was all that remained, as it was late in the season and they were closing the place the following day. Despite being well positioned, presiding over a black lake in its foreground, with a mountain top just behind it, the hotel was an old and rickety place that had seen its best days a long time ago. Houdini had once performed here and it was home, allegedly, to dozens of ghosts.

The night King stayed there, he had a troubling dream of his son being chased down endless corridors by a possessed firehose. It was bad enough to wake him up. His family were fast asleep. Disturbed, King went outside on the balcony for a smoke and looked at the eerily beautiful snow-capped mountain tops glistening a in the moonlight. By the time he finished his cigarette, the outline of *The Shining* had taken form in his brilliant mind.

I hired a car and drove up to the nearby Rockies with my friend Sheila, who I'd been working with in Denver. As part of the assignment, I went downstairs to meet the resident clairvoyant, a lovely lady who reminded me of Anjelica Huston but with silver hair. She read my fortune as a small artificial Christmas tree glowed in the corner of the room. It was May. She was quick to spot that I had Parkinson's even though no symptoms were presenting, and then she got on to the subject of my daughter. She told me Aggie would eventually get on a trial that would change a great deal for her for the better, repairing some of the damage done by her illness. It was all I needed to hear.

It's like the Greek myth of Pandora opening her box and unwittingly unleashing hell and letting everything from spite and hate escape into the world, with the last and only good thing to emerge being hope, a small ray of light that floated past her, and then disappeared. Sometimes hope gives us something to believe in in the face of nothing. Some days hope is all I have, but hearing this lady up in the Rockies with her rare talent telling me my daughter would one day benefit from being on a trial meant everything to me.

That night in the bothy at Camasunary, I felt isolated by my illness to the extent I didn't much feel like talking to Finn, Matt and Fergus. There was something really defeating about the self-admission that I could not survive without the drugs, and however much I hated taking them, I needed them to get through the day.

To the insistence and then delight of the school reunion gang, Fergus set up his sound bath drum, and he and Finn began to play it quietly – drum is definitely the wrong word; it sounds much more melodious than that. I went outside for a cigarette. It was so pitch black out there that I couldn't see my feet, nor even my hands. It was like being in a primal soup, as if I was suspended at the beginning of creation and I didn't know which way was up. Then a few minutes later a door opened in this third dimension and out stepped my son, now nineteen; tall, rangy with a face like Matt Dillon in the film *The Flamingo Kid*. He was all cheekbones and chin, brown eyes and thick upwardly angled eyebrows. But for all his handsome looks and thrift-store cool, he was very much a soulful character who thought deeply about life, philosophy, the planet and his part in it. He was sensitive. Sometimes I worried he thought about things a little too deeply, because there's a price to pay for that level of sensitivity, leaving yourself open to hurt.

He spotted the orange eye of my cigarette and as his night vision improved, he could see me leaning against the wall and came and leant beside me. The stars were appearing one after the other, and we began to see some of the constellations take form.

'We're all connected Dad, all of us, to this,' he gestured to the sky.

'I know,' I said, 'and once we start to trust that, life gets so much easier and more rewarding. The problem is, at least in my case, it's so easy to lose that trust when things start going wrong. Look what a mess I've made of my life,' I said.

'Sometimes things are meant to go wrong, so things that are right can take their place,' he said, sagely.

Albert Einstein is often said to have remarked, 'There are only two ways to live your life. One is as though nothing is a miracle. The other is as though everything is a miracle.' The happiest times we experience in ourselves are when we're unchained by our thoughts and able to be in the moment and look at life as if through a clear windscreen. I imagine the windscreen to be a bit like our perception, being hit by all the thoughts, like raindrops, constantly striking it. Rain is sloshing off the front windscreen until the window washer brushes it all off, and I think it's in just these tiny breaks between the rain of thought that everything is visible. That is when we feel free and have our insights; a little bit like the pause between two breaths. I think it's here that we begin to find the secrets of the universe because these moments, however brief, are those which reassure us there is a universal harmony which we are a part of and that things happen for a reason. However disconnected you may feel, events are taking place in your life right now, which in just a few years, or even months, you'll be able to look back on and truly understand why you were in this situation in the first place. And if you were, or are, at your lowest ebb, then this is exactly where you were (or are) supposed to be before you move on from it to a place of healing. We can only thrive once we've learnt the lesson.

The writer Henry Miller believed that it was only by hitting our rock-bottom that we could truly understand ourselves and our life, and the self-truths we are unconsciously running away from. Our redemption lies in sitting with it. 'When you surrender, the problem ceases to exist.

Try to solve it, or conquer it, and you only set up more resistance. I am very certain now that if I truly become what I wish to be, the burden will fall away.'

Miller goes on to say, 'The most difficult thing to admit and realise is that you alone control nothing. To be able to put yourself in tune or rhythm with the forces beyond, which are truly the operative ones, that is the task and the solution.'

Finn tossed the end of his rollie away. 'I don't tell you this often enough Dad, but I love you.' I was glad it was dark as he hugged me, I had tears streaming down my face.

That night my body shook like an ocean buoy in a ragged storm. I tried desperately to hold myself tight so my arms and legs weren't rattling on the wood surface that I was sleeping on, and so I wouldn't wake people up. From the movement of my vibrating arm and constant creaks coming from my part of the room, it sounded and looked like I was masturbating. With the absence of my sleeping pills, I spent most of the night wide awake, dreading the morning and all the walking and exercise that lay in wait for us the next day.

When morning finally came, I was so tired I felt like I was stoned and slightly paranoid. From the bothy window facing west was the most amazing panoramic view of the nearby bay and fine white sand beach, peeking out from arabesques of black seaweed. There were some big waves rolling in, crested in white foam, and, wasting no time, Matt and I were soon in it. I'd seen photos of Camasunary Bay, in sunshine, its shallows fired with patches of turquoise, but today the water was gun-grey and mean-looking.

From the sea, we had a fine view of the lush green meadow that stretched from the skirts of the mountain all the way to the shoreline. Prime grass explained why so many deer came to rut here. The season starts in September and finishes in November, and from the bothy it's possible to see an endless tournament of red deer stags, would-be champions, clashing and locking their horns in order to secure the right to mate. What an amazing place to battle your foe, I thought to myself. Could it be any more dramatic?

The place possessed a primal energy; there was something so raw and ancient about it. It seemed to earth my paranoia and settle my mind. We didn't waste any time getting changed. It was later in the day than I would have liked, and because I'd left my medication in the car on the other side of the mountain, because there was no way that I could endure another night of no sleep, we had to make the climb in daylight and find somewhere to sleep. The plan had been to leave here the following morning at about 5 a.m., when it was still dark, and then walk over the mountain again and head from Skye all the way to Inverness to catch a midday flight. It had been such a dangerous walk in the dark that it was a nonstarter even to think about doing it again.

I looked up at the sheer scale of the mountain that we had still to climb and the sharpness of the gradient.

I started thinking about getting stuck in the dark again and it put the fox among the chickens in my mind. 'Guys, we need to leave, now.'

Now that I knew we could summit and descend even in darkness, it didn't seem to take that long to get up the mountain and walk down the other side. Matt had carried Fergus's broken rucksack as well as the supply bag and his own rucksack, bearing it quietly and just getting on with it. However, I managed to fall over in the middle of a big puddle on the last 200 metres. What is it that happens with us on the last leg of a race? It's as if our bodies capitulate just before the finish line, even though it's within view.

Once at the jeep, we changed into blissfully dry clothes and fresh warm socks. It's the little things in life that make the difference to the bigger picture. Just knowing that we had made up our mind and we had a plan was all I needed to make me feel better. I counted our lucky stars; neither Fergus or myself had hurt ourselves when we fell, we had gotten a little decent footage and we had survived the drama of last night with everything intact. It made me think of something that Epictetus wrote. Epictetus, by the way, was neither an emperor nor a senator, he was a common slave and had a permanent limp where he had been beaten by his master. He truly knew and understood the meaning of the word *difficulty*.

'Every difficulty in life presents us with an opportunity to turn inward and to invoke our own inner resources. The trials we endure can and should introduce us to our strengths … Dig deeply. You possess strengths you might not realise you have.' Epictetus became one of the greatest Stoics. Seneca also writes on the theme of our getting to know ourselves and growing as a result of hardship, 'I judge you unfortunate because you have never lived through misfortune. You have passed through life without an opponent – no one can ever know what you are capable of, not even you.'

Up until last night, I had unconsciously defined the parameters of what I was physically capable of, which wasn't much these days. And though I hated every foot, yard and stone on that fucking mountain path, I nevertheless owed it a debt of gratitude, because it showed me that I still had the necessary minerals to climb it. Just. And my body, having had to redefine and widen its borders, would now have no excuse for cowering in the face of lesser quests.

When we reached Matt's house later that day, I gave my thanks to the gods for the little fire that was burning in their cosy front room with the Captain Nemo blue walls. Matt made up a blow-up bed for me on the floor, while Finn took the couch. It struck me how important it is to remember the contrasts in life. After the last couple of nights discomfort, tonight's set-up was splendid. I lay contentedly with the window open, a breeze coming in on one cheek and the warmth of the fire on the other.

I thought to myself, 'If I hadn't left my meds in the car, we could so easily have stayed another night at the bothy in Camasunary, and then we would have had to get up while it was still dark and climb the mountain. Plus, we would have had a mad race to get to the airport. It was as if everything happened as it was meant to happen – we just needed to trust in the process of it. I was more exhausted than I had been in a long time; I would pay for my walk and climb. We had achieved very little in terms of the work that we set out for ourselves for this weekend, but what we had learnt was a lesson, is that *in the presence of haste, how little gets done.*

I could feel the tightness in my calves and quads, and it was a good feeling. I took a sip of water, looked at the dying embers in the log-burner and at my sleeping son in the firelight, and then I fell in to perhaps the deepest of sleeps that I remember since developing this sleep-devouring disease.

Chapter 11

Loch Coruisk

It's the Journey that Matters

Most of us live in the Tomorrow, if we're really honest with ourselves. We tell ourselves things will be better when we're earning more money, or have more time; when we meet the right person, live in our dream home by the sea; when we have that car, or visit Kyoto in the spring when the cherry blossom explodes ... I could go on; we've all got different hopes for the future. But it's one thing having a goal to work towards, which is essential, as when we strive towards something important, we are at our most vital, but it's an entirely different thing to blindly hope things will change in the future without doing anything to realise your future dreams. I'll never go to Kyoto – in fact, the cherry blossom is blooming outside my window as I write, which means spring has landed in Japan too – unless I make a concerted effort and buy a ticket or gain a commission from a travel editor.

And then there's the Past, that crooked old house in which memories are filed, where we often find ourselves dwelling in the Nostalgia Room in which hangs a light bulb that rose-washes our recollections to make them seem so much better than the present. Deeper down in the basement is the Trauma Room, where bad experiences are kept boxed, under lock and key. It's here that we creep down to more than we should, masochistically feeding our mind old damaging memories that once cut us deeply and still hold us back.

The only place we have is now. This moment, right here in the present. None of us know what will happen in time to come, as it is not yet here, and it's our actions right now that determine what that future will look like. That doesn't mean you need to work your butt off and only relax when you get to the top of whatever tree you're climbing, as there's every chance you'll fall off or feel cheated once you finally get to the summit. But it means the seeds you plant today will partly determine what happens to you in the future.

The only truth is how you are feeling in the present, right now. Our level of aliveness comes from our ability to connect with the moment, to be alert to the things happening around us, and when we do manage to stop thinking forward and backwards in time, that is when we feel engaged with the world around us – whether it be to the place or the people in that place.

Switching off your thoughts is how you get present. For me, wild swimming is so immersive in the now because it demands your attention to the fact you are controlling your breathing in a chilly temperature, and you feel very much in your body as it is being subjected to such a rude awakening. And 'waking' is exactly what it is; nature's benign shock to your system that uproots you from negative spiralling thoughts as soon as you enter the water. As you first slide into this other world, you don't look at the opposite end of a loch and say, 'I'll be happy when I get there,' as after a few minutes' discomfort in this element that you spent nine months floating around unconsciously in before you were born, you are perfectly content and hyper present. Your skin tingles with the touch of water and your lungs feel like they are expanding as you settle into the discomfort. Welcome to the now.

It was an overcast morning in Elgol, the little fishing village crouched beneath a hill near the end of the Strathaird Peninsula, and the departure point for Loch Coruisk if you're travelling there by boat. The alternative is a 10-mile hike from Sligachan over steep terrain, the ledge of rock known as the 'Bad Step', and peaty bogland. As Finn and I waited on the stone jetty, Matt, our pathfinder, regaled us with local myths attached to the lake. 'Legend has it that this loch was the lair of a kelpie, a shapeshifting demon who appeared as a harmless black pony near the water's edge to draw children towards it, then dragged them down to the watery depths and feasted on their souls.'

'Nice,' said Finn, sparking up a rollie.

In just a few days of being away in Skye together, we felt as if our systems had been recharged. There was something so elemental and healing about the island; it was as if it was constantly working its magic on us.

Beside us on the ramp were barnacled lobster pots and a thickening knot of tourists. Beyond them, a perfect little crescent of sandy beach was strewn with boulders and seaweed. Matt scanned the horizon and pointed at a little craft puttering towards us. Its wooden galley and deck were a deep chestnut, and peering through the window beside the bearded face of the skipper was a border collie who looked like she was driving. Along the boat's white bough, a name read *Misty Isle*. A young lad with a pleasant face jumped off the boat on to the jetty and attached a thick mooring rope to a cleat. 'Welcome aboard,' he said.

'What else do you know about the loch we're heading to, Matt?' I asked as we climbed aboard.

'Turner painted it. It's one of the most dramatic places on the island.' Then he added, 'Oh, and there's supposed to be an *Uruisk*, a half-man half-goat creature that haunts it.'

'Along with the kelpies ...'

'Yes, it brings bad luck to anyone who sees it.'

As the boat cut through the milk-blue water of the sandy-bottomed shallows, it deepened to ink blue as the landmass fell away beneath us. Far off in the distance you could see the mountains of the Cuillin range. The rounder softer ones in the foreground were the Red Cuillin, while the taller jagged peaks glowering in the background stacked up against one another like rows of serrated shark's teeth, were the Black Cuillins.

'How deep is the lake?' asked Finn.

'Deep,' replied Matt. '100 metres in some places. And it's creepy as hell come nightfall, you may hear things in the dark.'

Matt is one of the most down-to-earth characters I have the pleasure of knowing; nothing seems to shake him. Nor does he subscribe to the paranormal – his mind is too methodical – but even he seemed slightly spooked.

'Think I'm more worried about the midges,' said Finn.

Misty Isle Boat Trips have been operating out of Elgol for three generations of MacKinnons, and father and son, respectively Sandy at the wheel, and Seumas Jr on the microphone, were present that morning. Seumas Jr had flame-red hair, an effortless charm and the ability to hold the attention of his captive audience – even the testosterone-dripping Dutch lads on tour, with their comedy kilts, were becalmed – as he related local legends and pointed out nearby islands, between passing around cups of hot chocolate.

'Believe it or not,' he said cheerfully, 'I am the descendant of John MacKinnon who carried "the lad who would be king", Bonnie Prince Charlie, to safety in 1746.'

I have always loved journeying by boat, the sense of progress you feel as you glance back at the dock you just left, which now lives in the past, and cast off towards your unseen destination, hidden in the future. Having done that, your eye submits to what is around you in your immediate vicinity: the water lapping at the bow; the voices and conversations of others; the breeze or chill on your cheeks; the wheeling of seagulls following your wake. You lean back against the gunwales, letting out an exhalation of simple contentment that comes from deep within you. It's as if you realise that you are powerless to go anywhere and so you submit to the now.

On a lucky day, you can spot puffins, porpoise and dolphin on the way to Loch Coruisk, but today we contented ourselves with a flock of black shags and a colony of grey seals. Like stranded overweight mermaids, they lay on ledges of rock, the boat passing sufficiently close for us to spot their babies with their long lashes and spotted coats. Ten minutes later, we moored up against a stone jetty, and as the other passengers alighted and climbed up the steep steps that led to the hidden loch, we grabbed our rucksacks and set off.

'Are you staying the night here?' called Seamus Jr after us.

'Yes,' I answered.

'Good luck.'

'Thanks.'

'We'll pick you up tomorrow at 1 p.m. ...

'Okay,' I said.

'Oh, and keep your eyes peeled for the goat-man.'

It was a short 300-metre walk to the freshwater loch, which turned a rich emerald green as the sun punched through the clouds on our arrival. Rising around the imposing lake at its northern tip, like a black fortress, were sheer walls of basalt, and enormous boulders of gabro rock, rough as a cat's tongue and to which your shoes stuck like glue.

For a few minutes, we skimmed stones, then Matt announced he was going ahead to set up camp. I looked down the loch's narrow but endlessly long expanse; it seemed to go on forever. 'How will we find you?'

'I'll be at the end of the lake, you won't be able to miss me. Keep an eye out for two orange tents.'

'How far is it?'

'Just follow the shoreline of the loch,' he replied, cryptically. 'There's a little beach at the tip.'

Then he was gone, fleet footed and moving across the wet rocks with the surety of a Chamois mountain goat.

Finn and I ate a couple of cold bacon sandwiches I'd brought along from breakfast, then we began to amble along the side of the lake, our attention focused on the slimy stones and rocks we were placing our feet amongst. My balance had been under siege from Parky lately, and it was a full-time job not falling over. I was so busy with this task that I began to ignore where I was, instead thinking impatiently about getting to the end of the walk.

It was hard going even on the sticky gabro rocks; the light turning to dusk as long shadows crept across the marshland. Finn and I took it in turns to pick a route through the bog boulders and stones, which sometimes ended in cul-de-sacs of water or mud into which our boots disappeared. And so we would have to pick our way back to our original waypoint.

Twilight was gathering in nooks and skerries as we reached the crest of a hill, confident it would reveal the end of the lake, as we had now been walking for hours on end. But to our disbelief, we discovered we were only halfway there. My mood dipped with my shrinking energy levels, 'How long *is* this bloody lake?' I asked in exasperation.

Finn patted me on the shoulder, his tanned face cracking a weary smile. 'We'll get there when we get there, Dad. Let's just enjoy the adventure.' He lifted off the straps of his rucksack and let it fall off his shoulders to the ground. It was getting cold. We sat and smoked a roll-up together in soulful silence, immersed in a kind of peacefulness; he was only nineteen, but his wisdom was that of an old soul. 'This is fun,' he said.

We sat there gazing at the rock formations of the walls enclosing the loch, spotting the faces of old crones and giant trolls. The last time I'd done this was in 2018, a few years before in Iceland. I'd been doing a story there on the remote north-east, where tours had just recently begun to go around the volcanic sites and places where lava had frozen in strange formations millions of years ago. The Icelanders believed these rocks that uncannily resemble faces are actually trolls which were caught out by the dawn light as they shuffled tardily to their lairs like unpunctual vampires. Instead of turning to ash, trolls simply freeze.

I'd stopped thinking of the finish line and how much I couldn't wait to lie down after some chow; I was here in the moment with one of my favourite people in the world, playing a game in an eerily beautiful location.

An hour later, the darkness thickening around us, the sheer basalt walls towering above us in a vast amphitheatre, we finally spotted two orange tents as a torch flickered within one. When we eventually got there, Matt had a fire burning and a pot of cooked chorizo and pasta on the go. It tasted delicious. We sat on our haunches and watched the stars appear in the night sky, the fire crackling, the sound of an unseen torrent high up in the rock face.

'This is just the sort of place you can imagine yourself looking at a star that suddenly moves and gets bigger and turns out to be a UFO hovering over the loch,' said Finn, thereby beginning a continual run of ghostly tales we kept going for hours until the whisky was gone and the fire was reduced to a few burning embers. I had to pinch myself at my good fortune; here I was in this beautiful, lonely place with my son and my good friend for company, and a freshwater lake in which to swim in the morning, not to mention a turquoise pool as clear as glass that fed into the northern tip of the loch just 50 yards away. Yes, my health was markedly worse in terms of tremor and dyskinesia than the last time I was on Skye, but so long as I was able to delight myself with these natural riches it was me who was winning, not the disease.

That night, the wind howled across the back of the tent, flapping the thin nylon and visiting my dreams with goat-men and red-eyed black ponies with seaweed manes. Outside the tent, I was awoken by something that screamed, perhaps the caw of a fish eagle, or maybe a frustrated kelpie.

Dawn touched our tents with dew, our bodies stiff with bad backs from sleeping on a hard surface. Half-asleep, we wandered the short distance to the beautiful pool Matt had talked of and slid into the brilliant turquoise water to wake up. I dived down to the bottom, happy as a nereid, and held on to a submerged rock so I could savour the underwater destination. The poem *Ithaca*, and one of its final verses came to mind: 'Ithaca gave you the marvellous journey. Without her you would never have set out. She has nothing left to give you now.'

'Circe's eye', the name with which I christened the pool, had been so much more than an emerald gem, a long walk capped off with a brief swim in crystalline water; it was the adventure to reach it and the great conversation that lubricated the hours that took us to get there, that I would best remember.

Chapter 12

Joining Up the Dots

For me, each time I go to Skye it feels a little bit more like home. I believe there are places in this life in which we feel more naturally relaxed than others. Some places just *feel* right. It can be an island, village or a nameless piece of land. Sometimes it may be the general layout of a place, a configuration of buildings and land which reminds us of a place we've felt happy in before which is similarly configured: farmhouses at the same angle, or fields behind. Other times, the feeling is stronger and it's as if it speaks to us that we can feel safe there. Perhaps we were here in another life, and depending on the urgency of how a place talks to us, we can tell if we lived there or whether we simply passed through and decided to spend a bit of time. It sounds a bit fantastical, but why not? Skye is like that for me.

When I think about the happiest travel moments I've experienced, all of them without exception have been on islands. My work trips and family holidays in Croatian and Greek islands, my visit to Kodiak Island and the sister islands of Martha's Vineyard and Nantucket. Then there's Iceland, right up there near the Arctic. And finally, domestically, the Scilly Isles and the Inner Hebridean Isles. I wonder why I prefer islands; is it because I'm surrounded by water and that makes me feel safer, or that I'm harder to reach, at some unconscious level? Or is it because I sailed to them in other lives?

And just as there are places that make us feel relaxed as if we've been there before, there are certain houses which cultivate a sense of calm and timelessness, too. I sometimes get this when I go to a particular bookshop in Hay-on-Wye, where reclining in the deep seat of a divan, I am perfectly placed to stay for the rest of the day (or the rest of my life!) without moving, as long as I have a book to read. The energy is just right. It's like being in the Goldilocks zone, but don't ask me what the exact criteria is; purposely, I haven't given it that much thought – it's really just a feeling of contentment.

I remember staying in Thailand on Ko Phi Phi Don, a little island which is close to its sibling Ko Phi Phi Lei, which is a nature reserve and was used as the desert island in the film *The Beach*. It was Christmas time, and there was this guy there at the hotel, and he had a big nose, perfect teeth, a large head and radiated a kind of cheesy glamour like some modern-day Dean Martin. It turned out he was a teacher, and I remember him quite specifically saying that he had no understanding why, but when he first arrived as a stranger in Kyoto in Japan, he knew that this was where he was going to live for the remainder of his life. 'It was as if my soul could breathe here,' he said. You may think it the most risky decision he'd ever made, but having straightened out his affairs in the US, he then went and opened up a language school for foreign students in Kyoto and never looked back. He described Kyoto as the round hole for his round peg, and he said he'd always been searching for a place which felt like home, but just hadn't found it until he got there.

I sometimes had the same feeling about Skye and pretty soon I was finding an excuse to come up here two or three times per year. But the problem with finding a place where you feel a sense of belonging is that it shines a light on everywhere else in comparison. While I loved the Cotswolds, I didn't feel I'd spilt my own blood there on a battlefield in a past life, nor did I feel I had made any great kinships other than my pals Hugh and Roger. And the rest of my friends lived in Warwick and in London, or in and around Brighton.

In Cirencester, it was as if I was always waiting for us to move again somewhere permanent and it all felt like a kind of rehearsal. And then my daughter was ill, as was I, and I didn't feel like I had the time or the energy to move anywhere else. Yet when I was on Skye, it was as if things made sense at a basic molecular level, like they'd been pared down to their simplest form. And while I knew that I couldn't spend the rest of my life wild swimming, it was one of the ways that life made more sense to me. Skye, a place where I could stop thinking and just be, where I didn't feel like I should be anyone or anywhere else. I consider myself extremely fortunate to have found even one place where I can do this.

Just as there are places in life that we feel we have known before, I believe there are also professions and cultures we feel drawn to, and yet we have no idea why. I don't know why, but I have always felt a predilection for all things nautical and American from the days of whaling. I hate whaling itself, just as I hope I would have hated it in its heyday when spermaceti oil was much sought after to light the desks of America and the world beyond. But for some reason I feel very familiar with this era and I have a feeling that in another life I worked on a whaling ship. I also love writing, that ancient discipline in which a smith hacks away at a rock face of infinite words and shapes, crafting something meaningful for others to read. I don't know why I'm drawn to this curious art, I just am.

I also think that there are times in our life when we are lucky enough to cross paths with people we have known in another time. And it's only after leaving their company and running into regular folk that you realise how very fine those people are, how comfortable you feel with them and the rarity of the connection that you share with them. For instance, my good friends Buddy Vanderhoop and his wife Lisa – a former National Geographic producer – who run a company that takes people fishing on Martha's

Vineyard. Almost as soon as I met them one golden morning in Menemsha in the south-west of the island, it was time to go home to my hotel. The day had passed so quickly, with such ease, as we sailed out to sea and later visited Buddy's mum who owned the seafood café by Gay Head lighthouse. I felt like I had been in the company of old friends. We hadn't stopped laughing and smiling all day. Was I extra relaxed after a busy week working in Boston teaching and trying unsuccessfully to keep still in front of a thousand people? Or had I met these people before and now we'd crossed paths again?

As I mentioned earlier, Buddy had a scrimshaw, an illustrated sperm whale's tooth. It had been engraved by his great-great uncle, Amos Smalley, who had killed a white bull sperm whale off the coast of the Azores. So, I had come to find out about one fish ('Jaws') for a newspaper and ended up finding out a whole lot more about another (the white whale).

I keep in touch with Buddy and Lisa, and know that if I was in trouble they would do their best to help me. And vice versa. That trip to Martha's was the inspiration for getting my own whale tattoo and the ultimate reason that I came to free dive with sperm whales in the Caribbean, writing a story on for the *Financial Times* a few years later.

I think of life as being like a series of dot-to dot pictures, and some pictures like the example above are easier to spot than others. I believe there is a celestial web that we cannot see and each of us is connected to one another through this interstitial grid of energy. When we start seeing the dots joining up, that is when we have started to trust the mystery of the universe and start acknowledging that events are indeed connected. It really helps you get through the black chaotic times because you're able to say to yourself, 'Okay, so this makes no sense to me now, but I'm going through this hardship for a reason and a couple of years down the line this will be just another dot in a series of many that will make up a constellation of sense; one with a happy outcome.'

Now, I don't blame you for thinking this is a load of tosh. So let's try and see if I can find an example of one such constellation. The easiest way to spot them is to focus on a really good thing that has happened to you and then look back on the events which preceded and caused it. Sometimes the spaces between dots can span many years, other times they are closer. Alongside your own efforts, certain other individuals will have been responsible for driving the event (the dot) to happen.

Okay, so let's say writing this book – which I hope will help others, whilst helping me understand the madness of the last fourteen years – is my 'good thing'. Looking back, many of my dots were teachers and though I have long forgotten the names of stodgy History teachers, I can clearly remember each of my English teachers. The first who noticed my writing was a guy called Mr Bowler, and I was about seven years old. The next teacher who spotted it was Mr Ivatt; I was eleven and he took the time to write to my parents to alert them to this talent. He was followed by Mr Duncan-Hill when I was thirteen. Then came Mr McAvoy, when I was sixteem, and after him Dr Derek Alsop, who taught me at degree level. Since then, there have been other sponsors of my writing, whether publishers, editors or literary agents.

At first the teachers said I was good at it, next that I was a natural, and then that I should do it for a living or that my writing was a talent that shouldn't be wasted. And now here I am writing books for a living. Between those obvious dots leading me forward have been more *evidential* dots which told me I was pushing in the right direction, doing the right thing. It might have been seeing my writing on the front page of the travel section of the *Daily Telegraph* or scooping a writing award for the *Sunday Times*, or writing a bestselling book with Tyson Fury; all of them represented 'evidence' that I was on the right track. My biggest evidential dot was writing a wellbeing blog for a bank, which was about feeling good and making the best of life. I had been diagnosed with Parky for about two years, and I realised through writing this blog that it was a joy to help and inspire others who I hadn't met. Since then, I've been sought out by people who my work resonates with and who want me to write their stories, and that means a hell of a lot to me.

Those dark, self-doubting days you may be experiencing right now are not much fun, but you have to go through them in order to slough off your old skin to reveal the bright new one underneath. Sometimes it might feel like you don't know what your direction is, but if you can try and lean into some of the good things that have happened to you in recent times and track them backwards, you may well find the beginnings of a dot-to-dot constellation that isn't fully realised yet, but will be soon enough.

The closer that we get to our inner selves, the more we are able to see where the dots connect, and understand that our feeling lost and depressed is just part of a transition period. It's you and life telling yourself what you don't want, so you can look at it and decide what would be better for you. Knowing what you don't want is essential to knowing and appreciating what you do want.

I believe in a brighter future. And just by looking for more positives and opportunities, and trusting that everything will be fine, and if it's not I'll handle it, that's a good place to meet the beginning of each day.

I recently heard something which stuck with me: 'Destiny doesn't do home visits.' In other words, it's all very well just waiting for change to happen in your life, but as well as asking the universe, you can do your bit to make it happen. And day-to-day life gets more satisfying if you know you're putting in the effort at your end by breaking down what you want into goals that you can pursue and achieve in digestible chunks. But I also think that occasionally you need to just be still and, in that stillness, be it in the middle of a freezing loch or walking up a hillside, you will start to see your dots appear.

Chapter 13

Echo Lake (Loch Sneosdal)
Quit While You're Ahead

It was mid-February, 2024, another grey day on Skye, and Finn, Matt and I were headed to a place the Viking called Echo Lake, far north in the Trotternish Peninsula. 'It's a bit of a hike,' he announced. Whenever the Viking says this, you know you're in for a right long walk.

Just for a change, it had been raining heavily. As we walked across the spongy surface of the ground, rainwater was sluicing darkly beneath our boots. We soon abandoned the slippery mud-sucking track in favour of the bracken and gorse, but it too was completely water-bound. It made for hard going. Finn was walking with his thoughts and Matt and I pressed on as the Viking tried to remember the route. Presently, we walked past a herd of cows who watched us defensively, their young calves clearly visible. According to the website 'killer cows', there are an average of eighty incidents a year in the UK involving people and cows; three of them fatal, and forty involving serious injury. We moved back to the path and kept on cautiously. Finally, we summited at a ridge by a pool with a set of rotten antlers poking out of the water.

'It's not this one,' Matt said, reading my mind.

The three of us had formed a bond and travelled well together, comfortable with each other's silences. When we spoke, it was because we wanted to. In the distance near the crest of the next hill, a flock of sheep waited on a level clearing with yet more bones scattered about it. I listened to the sound of my feet sloshing around and my breath. Pretty soon I had zoned out, just the rhythm of breath and the slosh-slosh of my footsteps remained. It was in this state of total emptiness that I had something of an insight.

'Everything is going to be alright.' It was my own voice and yet it wasn't; this one felt deeper than my every-day voice. It was surer of itself for a start, and absolute in its conviction. It simply said, 'Things are going to be fine.'

In early 2023, I had signed up for Deep Brain Stimulation (DBS), a procedure whereby a device is inserted into the body which sends out a pulse to the brain and massively reduces tremor. The brain is a hugely complex organ, but in the process of reducing trauma very often other symptoms are dealt with as well; for example, the Parkinson sweats. DBS is a last resort option for people with advanced Parkinson's. For me, my symptoms were spiralling out of control; the dyskinesia had infested my body like wild ivy and it constantly pulled me in different directions. The tremor had got worse too. I just couldn't keep still. Nor was I sleeping regularly, and I felt absolutely exhausted. It was deepest winter, and I felt like Parky was rushing me towards an abyss.

For the last three or four years leading up to the point in 2023 when my neurologist suggested deep brain stimulation as a possible treatment for Parky, I had been privately pursuing getting on a stem cell trial at Cambridge University. Ever since developing the disease in 2011, I had been sure that I would eventually be cured by stem cell research. Remember that at that point in time, the very idea that you could use 'reprogrammed' cells and get them to go where you wanted and to behave in the right way seemed the stuff of science-fiction.

Successful stem cell trials for Parky had taken place in Japan and Scandinavia and were due to happen next in Cambridge. Once I discovered the name of the doctor leading the British research study there, I was assiduous in keeping my name current in his mind; dropping him an email every three months. Originally, the study trial was supposed to take place in 2021, but the COVID-19 pandemic put paid to that. And then when it finally looked like happening, after a few false starts, it turned out I didn't meet the criteria for the test because I was now too old! Me, a forty-year-old, too old? Only I wasn't a spring chicken any longer, I was now fifty-four years old.

The problem with waiting for medical trials is that they are often delayed, and once you've had deep brain stimulation, it's impossible to get on a stem cell trial for

Parkinson's, as the DBS eases the symptoms of the disease for the better. I had been holding out against DBS for years because I was determined to get on a stem cell trial, because the stem cells would replace my brain's dead cells, while DBS would just help temper the symptoms. One was a possible cure, the other was a treatment.

The first human stem cell trial to treat Parkinson's took place at Kyoto University in Japan in 2018, and was hugely successful in using transplanted reprogrammed foetal mid-brain cells to replace dead dopamine producing cells in the brain. Dopamine is an athletic chemical produced by brain cells that helps carry messages from one area of the brain to another, as well as giving us energy. These cells become damaged, stop working and are lost over time for people who have Parkinson's, which results in slow movement. The brain cannot replace or repair these damaged cells, so once they're gone that's it, but stem cell treatment can replace them with new healthy cells. Despite opting for DBS, I still believe I will be on a stem cell trial in the next five years.

Once I had embraced the idea of wearing a device to calm down my symptoms, I was now in the unique position of choosing which device I would use. The reason for this was that Southmead Hospital in Bristol, in partnership with a company called Sparks, was pioneering devices which were smaller. Rather than the orthodox DBS machines which were fitted inside the chest like a pacemaker, with wires running up through the neck into the brain, Sparks' approach was to operate on the skull, excavate some bone and place the device inside a cavity in the person's head. It took less time in surgery, three-and-a-half hours as opposed to five, and Sparks was openly looking for candidates to try it. Tens of thousands of people have successfully undergone the DBS procedure and their lives have been much the better for it afterwards, with the tremor gone – DBS sends out an electrical pulse to override it – and often many of the other symptoms too. As I said, it's not a cure for Parkinson's, but a fantastic way of masking the symptoms using science. As soon as you turn off the implanted machine, its benefits become patently obvious, as your body instantly becomes a writhing, shaking mass. But provided you keep your device sufficiently charged twice a week, you need never turn it off, so you won't have to worry. Yes, you sometimes feel like a mobile phone that needs plugging in and charging, but you get used to it.

The application process to qualify for this treatment is long and drawn-out, involving a preliminary study to see if you're likely to benefit sufficiently from the treatment, then being asked questions by a psychiatrist who must decide if the operation might be too much for you psychologically. Finally, you have an in-depth brain scan to map exactly where the incisions will be made on your skull.

Having passed the tests, I was down on the list to have DBS, and since the skull-implanted device was new, I figured it wouldn't hurt to get the latest invention. To give you a little bit more detail, the surgery involved peeling back the skin on the top of my head, as you would grass turf in a garden, and then the precise cutting of my skull and the removal of a chunk so that it could accommodate the device. This initial incision would be performed by a robot, while the rest of the precision work would be carried out by a neurosurgeon. I would be the twenty-fifth person in the world to have trialled the operation; essentially, I was a guinea pig.

For some reason, I was more comfortable with the idea of a device in my skull than having it fitted in my chest. There were risks involved, as there are with any brain surgery, namely stroke, infection and a host of others I didn't bother listening to. The way I saw it, I didn't really have a choice; if I wanted a better life, I had to go ahead with the operation.

The more dead time I had on my hands to think about it, the worse the prospect of the surgery seemed. So I had timed this current trip to Skye to almost coincide with the brain surgery; I would have only a day between my last swim in the Scottish water and going under the knife.

For my side of the bargain, in order for the anaesthetic to work, it meant not having a cold or coming down with a chill, or getting ill before the op. Touch wood, apart from this bloody illness called Parky, I'm very rarely ill, perhaps once every three years. In the meantime, I would listen to my body as I always did and stay in the water for however long my system deemed okay.

Back in England, I had plenty of time to dwell on the negatives, and though I was good at putting a brave face on things, the nearer the operation drew, the more secretly worried I was becoming. Would the operation change my personality? Would the surgery leave my skull a series of bumps as a permanent reminder of the surgery? But here in Skye I was safe in the island's embrace, and though I knew the big day was happening very soon, the isle had a way of distracting me with its magic and my freewheeling conversations with my son and the Viking.

When somebody has to start fiddling around with your brain, that is when you know you're in trouble, but I had no option; my dyskinetic involuntary movements were now so unbearable I was constantly left feeling exhausted and could never keep still. Imagine boxing an invisible opponent every day of your life, and you're getting close to what extreme dyskinesia feels like. The tremor is more like a constant drum roll playing out uselessly in your limbs, and then perhaps the most hated of my symptoms were my sweats. It was as if I lived in my own super-sensitive climate, and it was difficult to be in even a slightly heated room, as within minutes I would have to leave and go outside in a T-shirt just to try and cool down. I had experienced this for the last couple of years – even on assignment in Iceland I had wandered around in a thin jumper – but now the sweating, which thankfully had no odour, was happening every day.

Most recently, I'd had to go to London to meet and

have dinner with the legendary ten-times World jiujitsu champion, Roger Gracie. I was early for a change, and sat in the busy confines of the restaurant trying to think cooling thoughts of icebergs as my system overheated, while I broke into a typically inconvenient sweat which had me wanting to change my now wet T-shirt. Add to this that my hands were also shaking, and as soon as Roger and his friend Nina arrived, my dyskinesia played havoc under the table so I kept having to apologise to each in turn and reassure them I was sorry to keep touching their legs with my own, and that I wasn't playing footsie on purpose! My serviette was soon soaked in sweat and the entire contents of the water bottle were inside my bladder. And we'd barely started.

'I've got Parkinson's,' I said apologetically, 'but don't worry, by the time we work together, should we choose to, I'm hoping these sweats will have improved and that my shaky legs and hands will be still after my brain surgery next month.'

They were utterly charming as I did my best to chat with Nina and Roger about what has become the number one martial art in this country, namely Brazilian jiujitsu, all the time sweating and playing accidental footsie with them. Ordinarily I would have loved eating a first class dinner in the company of the GOAT (Greatest Of all Time) practitioner of jiujitsu, but all I wanted to do was head for the door. It was a difficult meeting to get through, and so, thoroughly deflated, on the bus back home I wrote and apologised to my literary agent and his assistant for wasting everybody's time, including theirs and most definitely Roger and Nina's. Life at times was becoming so challenging, I didn't know if I had much grit left in me to fight this disease.

But tramping through those wet fields past the grumpy West Highland cows, the sky pregnant with rain, I heard the voice inside me, the voice of me, telling me not to worry, it was all going to be fine and the operation would be successful. Just then we walked over a ridge and beheld the dark glory of Echo Lake. It was enormous and at one end a black cliff ran up to the clouds like a gothic bedhead (a bit like the wall in *Game of Thrones*, but the colour of embers). I remained in this state of elation for a short time. I couldn't care less that the weather was bad, nor was I worried about my imminent surgery, I'd been hooked up for a one-to-one with my deeper self, in turn a member of the universe, and it had given me the thumbs up.

It is when you learn to really switch into the present moment that things start feeling as if they make sense. Many of you will already have experienced this throughout your life. Like when you've written something you're really proud of that seemed to come from nowhere, but you know it was you that created it. Maybe it was something you painted; you were caught up in its creating and nothing else seemed to matter while you were doing it. It's like an inner flow of energy where everything just lines up. You don't know why exactly, but whatever it is you did, it was perfect. And it's not just the thing that you created, rather it's the moment in which you savour it that's the best. Everything is just right, and you have all you need. This is called 'being in the flow', and it happens when there's just the right amount of high challenge versus your skill level, and you feel 100 per cent engaged in the pursuit; when everything is going right and nothing distracts your laser-like focus. Sportspeople also call it being 'in the zone'.

The term 'being in the flow' was coined by psychiatrist Mihaly Csikszentmihalyi (prounounced *chick-sent-me-hiy-ali*), who took on the unenviable task of finding what makes people happy, and the meaning of life. He discovered that doing what you love leads to generating meaning and happiness in your life. And this happiness comes only from within, never from exterior influences. His study subjects were paged randomly at any time and asked to write down what they were doing and the feelings that their activity produced. The happiest moments weren't caused by chance, but rather when a specific activity was enjoyed. These activities that we have a passion for have the power to banish thoughts of worry or anxiety; Csikszentmihalyi refers to them as 'flow'.

According to him, flow is a place where you stop think-ing and just do. It's an optimal experience which gives us a sense of satisfaction because we are creating some kind of order. And after each experience the person feels closer to themselves than they were before. Put plainly, it gives us happiness and a sense of meaning in life – whatever is meaningful to the individual – and it gifts us self-knowledge and a purpose.

It's an elevated state. Perhaps you experienced this feeling on the rugby pitch as a teenager; a particular try that you scored, as you swept past the first person and then dummied the second, your legs seeming possessed of an energy which they didn't usually have. It was a time you reached into yourself and pulled out something truly special, something you wouldn't ordinarily do, or an extreme to which you ordinarily wouldn't push yourself. Whatever it was, you seemed to have ability to slow time, to really understand what you were doing and execute it perfectly. The next thing you knew people were roaring, clapping you on the shoulder. This special moment was created by you.

I believe this level of satisfaction comes when you feel at peace inside yourself and with the external world. When you are maximising your potential. The writer Colin Wilson wrote about the state of flow, calling it a 'peak experience'. He himself had experienced these special moments – when his brain was flooded with consciousness and hope – numerous times in his life. But the first time he actually remembered having it was when he was lost in himself as a young man working as a lab assistant. He felt that his life was so dull that he had no place being in it. A little dramatic, but he resolved to kill himself, and without further ado went to the storeroom at the back of the chemistry lab and took a bottle of cyanide from the shelf, unscrewing the lid, lifting it to his lips and beginning to tip the bottle.

Just as the liquid was flowing, a voice within him told him very clearly to 'stop!' and he had a sense that there were now two people in the room; one was Colin Wilson, whom he thought rather silly, and the other was the higher being in himself, who possessed wisdom and calm and radiated a sense of equanimity. Just like the one who told me everything would be alright when I was walking to Echo Lake. Through this other self, the young Wilson felt suddenly connected to everything and for the next couple of days mundane objects and experiences appeared that much more wondrous and imbued with meaning, almost like nature's intense colours popping under the darkness of a pre-storm thundercloud. Details of leaves and trees made themselves known to him, and more importantly he had a sense of control over himself, and felt strangely calm.

When we find ourselves suddenly in a crisis in which our life is threatened, it can sharply wake us from a life that has largely felt like a long and dreary dream. The crisis puts us in such immediate danger it's no longer sufficient to just sit there; we are forced to do something. If we rise to the challenge of the crisis and survive, it rewards us with something special. Insight. Graham Greene had it as a youth when he very nearly shot himself in his back garden playing Russian roulette, just as Dostoevsky experienced this sudden waking up when he was in front of a firing range on the point of being shot, but was then exempted and sent instead to Siberia.

The scientist Abraham Maslow, rather than studying and working with people who suffered chronic depression or some kind of mental illness, chose a different approach to his subjects; he decided to work with people who were healthy. He discovered that mentally healthy people had peak experiences ('peakers') and generally felt more at one with the world, as compared to depressed people who saw things very narrowly and operated from the worm's eye view. That's because their depression wouldn't allow them to galvanise themselves and rise up above their problems. Imagine when you're up against it. We've all been there, when everything feels like it's crowding in on you like when Princess Leia, Luke and Solo get trapped in the trash compactor in *Star Wars*. It's when the walls are closing in that you have to rise and look down with a bird's eye view, objectively seeing the problem for what it is, and then going back down to address it.

Healthy, happy people believe in moments of bliss because they've experienced them already. Maslow also discovered that people who possessed a positive nature were more likely to feel that rather than being an orphan of the world – they belonged to a huge universal family. Peakers don't believe the world is out to get them. The existentialist, Jean-Paul Sartre lived and wrote in the dangerous days of the Second World War and was part of the French Resistance. In later years he would look back on this time as the period when he felt most alive; life was perilous and the Nazis could have discovered his involvement with the Resistance at any time. He lived on his wits and nerves, and felt he was part of something with a bigger meaning than himself.

Wilson says that it's when we are on 'all systems go' that we are at our best, but as soon as we are safe and comfortable, we become bored, our energy drops and we are no longer happy. Forty-nine per cent of us is the essence of who we really are, and 51 per cent of us is a robot that tries to take over everything we do consciously; from driving the car to having a conversation and having a shave. The more that we allow our inner computer to take over, the less involved in our own lives we are. But the good news is that it doesn't take much effort and positivity to change the balance from 49 per cent to 51 per cent so we're feeling more electrified by life. Then it's more like we're living it, not it living us.

Once Maslow's students identified what peak experiences were – moments of intense connectedness, bliss and peace – they began having them more and more often, almost like training a magical muscle. Peak experiences come and go at their own whim. Wilson devoted a large part of his life to trying to invoke and control these special moments, and found that when he was particularly tired, that was the time when his mind was most open to suggestion. He could either allow his negative brain to take over, or he could will the blossoming expression of a peak experience.

Wild swimming in water so cold it gives you a temporary gender reassignment – sending your balls back into your body – rewards you with the same release of happy chemical as if you had just had a narrow scrape with danger, but on a spiritual level it also resets your factory settings so that pages previously graffitied with unhelpful thoughts are for a limited time blank once more.

While Finn sent the drone camera for a run, I sat among the gorse on the sharp banks of Echo Lake and decided against going into its black expanse. In the fading light, the water was the colour of coal and it looked as tempting as a punch in the face. Something in my gut told me not to bother going in, and that I would catch a chill which would then mean I couldn't be operated on, and this surgery would then have to wait another month. The Viking concurred. So, instead, we played 'Echo!', our voices resounding off the black basalt cliffs. I took great pleasure in saying, 'Fuck you Parkinsons!' And hearing it echo again and again.

'Imagine if this cliff was a sleeping giant we just woke up with our echoes,' said Finn, bringing the drone home and landing it beside him. As I turned to watch him packing up his film kit and we started the long walk back from Echo Lake to the jeep, I reflected that during my illness he had grown into a fine man.

Chapter 14

Canadian Death Lake

Facing Fear

The difference between courage and bravery is that, where bravery is concerned, you're prepared for what lies ahead. Whereas for me courage is when you know what you're up against but you choose to go through it anyway, even though there's a good chance that the danger ahead may bring you down. It's about facing difficult odds but going for it anyway.

Matt and Finn call it the Canadian Death Lake because with its autumnal aspect of maple trees and oaks, and the snow-capped mountains in the background, something about is reminiscent of Canada. That's the Canadian explanation, the death bit is because when you swim in it – and it's super deep – it feels as if there's a malignance to the loch, like it doesn't want to let you get out. Certainly, it is the coldest water I have ever swum in; when compared with this forbidding, freezing loch, the glacially cold healing pool of Loch Shianta seems even more benevolent and welcoming. What you experience in the Canadian Death Lake is cold on a level I've only come close to once before, swimming in Bodo harbour in Arctic Norway; in real time it eats its way up your legs, past your calves and up your thighs; meanwhile it's working its way through your fingers and up your arms. You've literally got seconds – that's what it feels like – before your whole body packs up, not to mention the fact that your heart is beating so quickly.

Spending time in the darkness of the Canadian Death Lake actually feels like it doesn't do you any good, but because it is the last stretch of water before Inverness Airport, we always find ourselves going in for a quick dip before we return to our separate lives. And we all like to scare ourselves a bit, don't we? As you're front-crawling and your face goes under, there isn't anything but red water, which immediately turns into fathomless blackness all around you when your face is looking down. It's lonely and frightening. I feel as if this is a nightmare rendition of hell. If hell existed, it wouldn't be a place of burning towers, fiery-tongued devils and pug-like demons poking you in the behind with sharp little pitchforks; no, we'll leave the dramatic renditions to Hieronymus Bosch. Instead I imagine it to be the Canadian Death Lake, a place of utter darkness where you feel an impending sense of doom that grows until it screams silently in your ears as you paddle through an eternity of blackness.

We know when our time is up, I'm sure of it. Vikings believed that if they were lucky, they would be killed in the fury of battle, and winged female spirits called Valkyries would scoop them up and transport their souls to Valhalla. Here, all the great warriors got to sit at the table with Odin, the war god. It was the Viking version of heaven, or the equivalent to the ancient Greeks' Elysian Fields.

That said, if your number is called on a particular day, it's set in stone – it could be the number 33 bus that runs you over, or perhaps you fall and hit your head, but if it's your time there's no getting away from it.

Five years ago, while surfing in north Devon, I caught a rip-tide with the intention of leaving the rocks behind and getting out the back to the big waves. That day the sea was a strange menace, the current which usually flows south and makes you drift *down* the beach was headed in the other direction, pushing surfers against the rocks on the point. The waves were very big, but gloopy and unrideable, and as the rip took me into the impact zone of where the waves hit blade-sharp rocks beneath the water, I was pinned down by the current. There's no quicker way to tire yourself out than on a surfboard battling against waves as you try and escape them whilst also fighting a current.

For 20 very hairy minutes I tried to adapt to the situation, calmly thinking my way out of it; I tried to surf a few waves in, but I was effectively surfing inches above the rocks and heading straight for the cliff where they were breaking. After a few attempts, I was losing the battle to paddle out of the impact zone, my now exhausted arms sluggish as lead pipes. Next, I tried to punch out the back of the waves coming steadily at me by Eskimo-rolling as the wave hit me so it didn't drag me with it back to the rocks. The tide had come right in, and I could see my pals watching anxiously from the nearby shoreline and waving. Eventually, there was a break in the sets of waves and I paddled out across the rip and followed a smallish wave in. A moment later I was spat on to the beach.

My friends clapped me on the back and joked how close I'd been. Now I was safe, they could all go back to their chalets. One friend in particular waited till everybody had gone and quietly asked me in all seriousness, 'Rich, have you got a death-wish?'

'A death-wish?' I asked as I dried off. 'Why do you say that?'

'Because of what you are dealing with at the moment, it's too much for one person, what with you and Aggie. And you were the only one out on those waves, and you didn't stand a chance, yet you looked like you were almost enjoying it.'

'One thing I've learnt with mine and my daughter's illness pal, is how much I prize life; because when you're ill you never know how long you've got left, right? That's not to say I'm profligate about it, but I just realise that it is not going to last for ever and to make the most of it. So no, I don't have a death-wish.'

What is interesting is that for the whole of that 20 minutes' skirmish with the sea, I never felt like it was the end; I never stopped fighting for a way out of that watery trap. I believe we all know when it is our time, and until that hour we must 'not go gentle into that good night', but as Dylan Thomas tells us, 'Rage, rage against the dying of the light.' I don't mean literally rage, and I don't think Dylan did either – in your eighties or nineties you should aim to be mellifluous and gentle; not a crabby pain in the arse who everyone fears getting stuck in a lift with. I think he's telling us not to submit to the default setting of old age and instead to make the most of every day. As Ollie Ollerton wrote in his book *Battle Ready*: 'How old do we have to get before we understand that life is not supposed to be a punishment? And that we have keys to open the cage we've unwittingly built for ourselves.' The truth is that just as we can be lonely in a room full of people, equally we can be dying in the full blossom of youth if we are not making the most of our lives, doing what we love, being with the right partner who we nourish and, likewise, doing things which stretch us and make us happy.

Death doesn't walk a million miles to fetch you, it has been with you all the time. Every day you are moving closer towards your final appointment, whatever your age. Culturally, we're not brilliant with death in the West as compared with the East. In Vietnam, you are constantly thinking about your relatives who have passed because part of your rice field's income is dedicated to upholding their shrines. It's called ancestor worship. In Mexico, on 1 November, they celebrate the Day of the Dead. The deceased are toasted and celebrated, their photos come out, and graveyards up and down the country are lively with processions and partying by families next to their dead ones' graves. Death should not be something feared; anaemic, swept under the carpet, ever present and slyly watching us, like the chimes of an old Victorian clock echoing eerily in an empty house, Death is a quintessential part of life.

The Stoics made it their business to never forget the nearby presence of death. They had a term just to remind them, it was *memento mori* which roughly translates as 'remember you're dying'. In other words, don't take life for granted and don't, whatever you do, sleepwalk until your last days and only then realise that you've wasted your life. It's much too late by then. By reminding yourself of the closeness of death, you are inadvertently celebrating life and bringing it to the forefront, rather than taking it for granted.

You can buy medallions inscribed with 'memento mori' online at Etsy or the Daily Stoic. They're small enough to keep in your pocket, or wear about your neck, so just by feeling or seeing them, it reminds you that every day is a blessing.

When it is your moment, there's nothing to be afraid of. Whether your death is a violent or a peaceful one, I think the moment you cross is peaceful. Personally, I think death's hand will be a soft one, however hard the path might have been to meeting it. Death in itself is just another stage, the next adventure. There are many kinds of death in our life: the closing doors of relationships, of friendships and lovers; the sloughing off of old skins and seasons. We should learn from these that nothing is permanent, in preparation for our last breath, the final one at death.

There comes a point in old age where life loses its appeal because the body is in such poor shape that it makes doing anything an immense effort, and even going to the shops can seem like you're planning a foreign military campaign. I guess it's the same with the advanced infirmity of degenerative illnesses; death is very welcome. The mind might still be sharp, but the body is on strike. I think death can be an old friend to us if we meet it at the right time of our life when we're ready to go; and if it comes before, perhaps it is because we are required somewhere else or by someone who desperately needs us in another life.

Typically, when I talk to Matt on the subject of death, he is brutally pragmatic, 'I just think when the neurons stop firing and we stop breathing, there is nothing is left.'

Going back to *sympatheia*, the idea that all living things are interconnected, from eco-systems to humans, and therefore have an affinity with each other because we are all part of a larger organism, it reminds me of *The Time of Your Life*, a play by William Saroyan. He writes: 'Remember that every man is a variation of yourself. No man's guilt is not yours, nor is any man's innocence a thing apart. Despise evil and ungodliness, but not men of ungodliness or evil. These, understand.'

When we look on another human being as our brother or sister, we should not look to find faults in them, but try to help them where possible, and to understand that in the struggle that is life, some fall on hard times which bring out the worst in them.

Saroyan tells us to place the least value in 'matter and in flesh', for 'these are things' – like pride and vanity – 'that hold death and must pass away'. Instead, we should 'discover in all things that which shines and is beyond corruption'. Each of us, he believes, is a cup bearer of light, and he exhorts us that 'In the time of your life, live – so that in that wondrous time you should not add to the misery and sorrow of the world, but shall smile to the infinite delight and mystery of it.'

Marcus Aurelius also believes that we were not born to be alone: 'Human beings have been made for the sake of one another. Teach them or endure them.' Have sympathy for your fellow man.

Science is beginning to spot the neuro nuances in people and how this affects how differently we each see the world, through our own lens. What we all have in common is that we all experience fear, some of us throughout our day, others less so.

Healthy fear is a very useful ally to have on your side as it keeps you safe; like avoiding walking on the edge of cliffs, feeding lions or staring at a man with spiderwebs tattooed all over his face. Okay, we can probably replace the word 'fear' with 'common sense'.

There is a mountain in Skye's Cuillin peaks called Sgùrr nan Gillean (the peak of the young men) and Matt the Viking has tried to climb it twice. Each time he has been close to summiting the island's most famous Munro (a mountain over 3,000 feet), his common sense has told him today is not the day, be it because the snow has turned to ice and the gradient is so tricky and slippery, or because the people who are ahead of him on the slopes, keeping him company, have disappeared leaving him exposed and prey to his thoughts. Whatever, it niggles him that he has not yet climbed it (it would help matters if he didn't insist on there being snow on it at the time of his climb). Matt is listening to the millions of neurons in his stomach – each of us has a gut that possesses more brainpower than the average cat – that are feeding his brain with instinctive information from the gut. That's why it is so powerful and so often correct; we're kept alive by common sense, gut instinct and fight or flight fear.

We have naturally inbuilt fears, like fear of the dark, fear of the unknown and fear of death, all of which are there to protect us. But anxiety, which is a kind of fear of what may happen but rarely does, is different and does you absolutely no favours. It certainly doesn't protect you, instead it holds you back. And it's just plain exhausting.

Anxiety is what society feeds itself on, and it reminds me of the snake that slowly cannibalises itself from the tail up. It knows what it is doing to itself, but it just doesn't stop. Now, I don't know whether it's because of social media filling us with chronic self-doubt – the continual loom-ing presence of a Third World War, a rapidly warming planet or that the speed of life has become too quick for us to keep up, with tech that has overwhelmed us and left us behind, fearful of the new wave of AI – but anxiety is weirdly common these days. And anxiety is definitely not something we need to have around us.

Cortisol is the stress chemical that the amygdala, the lizard part of the brain, releases when we opt for flight rather than fight. Testosterone is what we produce more of when we go into fight mode. Unlike animals, who have an inbuilt mechanism to shake off stress and reset their nervous system (look at any wildlife documentary with a gazelle who has just made it out of the maws of a cheetah, the first thing they do is physically shake it off), humans often retain high levels of stress without realising it. We carry it in the stiffness of our joints, in our organs and posture, and we lubricate and marinate it in our uncon-scious thoughts. And unless we are aware of the stress levels we're trying to live with as if they are normal, and do something about, it can lead to panic attacks.

The quickest way that I know to get rid of a panic is to abandon the mind, or more precisely, the thinking that is creating and feeding it. Nothing does this better and more immediately than immersing yourself in cold water, but it's unlikely you are going to be having a panic attack near water or when you happen to be in your swimming gear. Better then to have a cold shower. And on your way to the shower ask yourself for some proof to back up why you are so anxious.

Q.1 Is anybody coming to harm me right now (hopefully the answer is no)?

Q.2 Am I dying right now? The answer is no.

Q.3 Am I running out of breath? The answer is no, you just need to breathe deeply.

The last two questions relate directly to your body, so you need to ask it for proof. So if none of the above are happening to you, you have everything that you need to survive right now. Of course, this is easier said than done, especially if you are in the tightening grip of a panic attack. But breathing slowly, and gently applying reason to your skewed thoughts is one way to deal with it. In the event that there isn't a shower available nearby, head for the bathroom anyway and fill the sink with cold water. Then, after a breath, place your head under water in the stillness.

I've experienced one panic attack in my life and it went on for almost two days. A summer ago, I was in Swansea seeing my sister, and gradually, over the course of the day this feeling of discombobulation grew and grew until it was big enough to wrap its arms around me and start playing with my mind. I'd run out of some of my meds; my happy pills which I need to take to balance me, because with Parky I no longer naturally produce dopamine, the body's energiser and one of its 'feel-good' chemicals.

I kept saying to my sis, 'I know what is going on here, I'm not scared, I just feel a bit weird.' This feeling a bit weird had gone out of control within a few hours and I was now experiencing a fluttering heartbeat and an advanced number of beats per minute that could have put the Happy Mondays to shame. After not getting any better over the course of the day, I opted to go to A&E.

'Try not to act mad,' I told myself.

I'm not mad, I replied to myself.

'Tell that to the ambulance driver over there who is watching you and pretending not to.'

As I looked over at a bearded chap, he pretended to look over my head.

I really don't want to end up in the loony bin.

'Try and keep still then, you're like an intoxicated gibbon.'

It just got worse from then on. My sister Lou was amazing; she humoured me, stayed with me and waited some 18 hours before we were finally seen by a doctor after midday the next day. By which time I hadn't taken any happy pills for four days, and I was leaping about with dyskinesia, acutely paranoid, my eyes wide and unblinking. The doctor who saw me was a young lady from the Philippines, who smiled and said, 'The reason you are having this feeling is you are suffering from withdrawal of your meds, nothing else.'

'So I'm not going crazy?'

'*Crazy?*' she said dismissively. 'Not at all. You're tired and you need sleep and rest.'

Astonishingly, this hospital business occurred just two days before coming to Skye. I had a day in bed, and gradually my marbles rolled back into their position. Touch wood, but I have never had a panic attack since. What restorative powers this island must have, because there I felt anything but mad. Rather, I felt rooted and earthed to this special place.

Chapter 15

Finding Hope for the Future

The lady at Inverness Airport check-in desk informed Finn and I that we were too late to check in. This was a problem. We had to get back as the day after tomorrow I was due to have surgery at Bristol hospital, having my head sliced open by a robot, for a neurosurgeon to insert a device just above my brain which would hopefully have a positive effect on the many different symptoms I was experiencing from Parkinson's.

The check-in lady must have seen the panic in my eyes, or noted the fact that my right hand was shaking uncontrollably, because she softened and said, 'Go check your bags in, you've got just enough time.'

After saying goodbye to Matt and Fergus, we rushed through security and flew back to Bristol that afternoon.

Earlier, while chatting with Fergus on the subject of why Kodiak bears are sometimes bigger than grizzly bears, I had what I can only describe as a 'Parky fit' while sitting in the Nemo blue lounge at Matt's house. I felt so comfortable with Fergus and his mum Michelle, I didn't even try and stop it. I was tired of trying to hold myself together all the time. My whole body was now in spasm, an inglorious mix of tremor and dyskinesia. My arms were flying all over the place, and the trunk of my body was shaking too. As were my teeth and bottom jaw. All I could mumble under my breath while smiling, was, 'Roll on Wednesday'. The day of the surgery, the day after tomorrow.

It was a hellish flight back to Bristol as chronic dyskinesia kept me in its grasp and never let me go until late that night. At 6 foot 1 inch, I'm not easy to hide in a plane and the extreme involuntary rapid jerky movements firing from my body every few seconds were quickly causing looks of concern. Just to make myself even more self-conscious, I also developed one of my famous sweats. I willed myself still with my eyes shut, but it only lasted for a few seconds. It was too violent to stop it with thought and meds alone.

Finn drove me back from the airport and dropped me off in Herefordshire before heading back to Cirencester. We had got on brilliantly and I hated seeing him go. What I hated even more was the prospect of not seeing my son or my daughter for the next six weeks, which is how long I was banned from driving whilst my brain recovered from its trauma. That evening my sister travelled up from Swansea to take me to my operation the following day. I couldn't drive there, as I had to turn up without any drugs in my system and abide by nil by mouth. It wasn't exactly fear I felt when I thought of the imminent three-hour operation, although there was definitely some of that, but more a kind of grim fatalism; if it worked, brilliant, I could start my life again. If it didn't, if something went wrong during the operation and I died, then that was supposed to happen too. I saw the procedure as a huge positive, a last chance. I just hoped turning my scalp into a building site would be worth it. And that, finally, I might get a good night's sleep.

On the day of my operation at Bristol Hospital, I changed into a medical robe shortly before the procedure and in the company of my sister I waited to be taken to the operating theatre. Getting to this point had been a fourteen-year journey of self-discovery I wouldn't wish on anyone. Had I learnt a lot about myself? I think so. I never believed I could drop so low, nor that I could lose sight of who I was and what really mattered to me. I also witnessed within me a refusal to give up and that even with the smallest chinks of light still glowing in my darkness, there was and still is *always* something to hope for.

The gift of stillness is something you cannot prize enough, unless you have played Richard Burton on stage who mesmerised you by hardly moving, or if you have your stillness taken away. The first thing I noticed as I gradually awoke from the anaesthetic was how still I was. Then, as my blurred vision began to focus in on things,

I noticed my sister sitting at my bedside. She smiled at me and held my hand. 'You okay, bro?'

It felt like a benign dream.

'I'm fine … I think.'

There were tears in her eyes. 'You are so brave going through this.'

I think I was crying too. 'I'm really not, Lou,' I mumbled, 'just didn't have a choice but to have it.'

I touched my fingers to my head and felt the bumps and pronounced features of the device now installed in my skull. It felt huge and invasive. The stitches were many and there were clots of blood in my hair but I didn't care, I was as still as a rock at the bottom of a Scottish loch. And they hadn't even turned the machine on yet; that wouldn't be for another couple of weeks. The surgeon had told me that the placebo effect could often make positive strides before the machine started working its magic, and as we know in my case, a bit of placebo goes a long way, as neither my hands nor feet were doing anything untoward. It was a joy to just lie there and hear my breathing rather than the percussive strokes of my tremor.

The benefits of the device continued throughout the night, as for the first time in eight years I slept a deep, dreamless sleep and felt truly recharged the following morning. I can't tell you how special it was, the fight and strength even after one night returning to my body. This was more like it! Now I had a chance again, a more level playing field. On the second day I woke to the loving presence of not only my sister but also my son. Finn ignored my stitched up head and looked at me with concern, 'You okay, dude?'

This was quickly followed by two of my best pals who had dropped everything to come and see me. One of them had brought me a film magazine, the other the latest copy of *New Scientist*. They were upbeat and kept pointing my attention back to my stillness. I longed to see Aggie again and sit beside her, stroking her hair, holding her hand, with her looking over at me, laughing at the ugly bumps and stitches in my head that made me look like Frankenstein. But she already spent enough time in hospitals, being checked on and monitored; she didn't need to be in another one now.

Over the next few weeks, the machine was switched on, and as it did I felt a wave of electric pulses shoot through the device in my head, and as my slightly shaking hands suddenly ceased all movement, I began to experience the miracle of deep brain stimulation.

At first I had no signs of dyskinesia whatsoever; in fact most of the time you couldn't tell that I even had the disease anymore. But the higher I jacked up the amplifyng pulse, the worse my dyskinesia and the more it affected my gait, which pre-surgery had been okay. It was a question of calibrating it just right – kill the tremor entirely with an excessively high pulse and it took away from my balance or smoothness of gait; get it just right and it affected neither and just about removed most of the tremor. What a small price to pay for what was no less than a second chance at life I was being given.

It was April, six weeks after the operation, and I was finally allowed to drive and go swimming again. I took my first post-op dip in the river Teme which passes beneath the towering ruins of Ludlow Castle. Foolhardy, perhaps, but I had not told anyone of my intention to swim in the river that morning; I didn't want to be talked out of it. It had been raining a lot these past few days and the current looked strong and full of vim as it ran past my feet green and silent. I eased my skin into the river and howled with its freezing sting, and although I could feel the ice water on my recently sealed scalp, its teeth exploring my scars, it was so wonderful to be in the water again, losing my breath and feeling the tingle of my skin coming alive once more. I didn't feel as if I was just swimming in a river, instead I felt in the midst of life in the eddies and currents of the present. And then, though my arms felt weak from inertia these last six weeks, I began to swim upstream, with something like a smile on my face.

Epilogue

My favourite part of the week? Sitting on the couch with my girl on a Sunday afternoon watching TV, Aggie holding my hand tightly. During that year when Finny wasn't talking to me, I still used to come and see Aggs at the family home. We would go out for walks, with me pushing Aggs in her wheelchair, or we'd sit on the couch and watch movies together. She would hold my hand, but as soon as she heard her mum coming down the corridor she would let go of it. As I said, she's smart as hell!

Agatha is now fifteen and the most inspiring soul I have ever met. It's a privilege to call her my daughter; her ability to smile, her indomitable spirit and her wicked sense of fun keep her afloat in the face of challenges no one her age should have to face. She has the most wonderful group of friends who adore her, the most fiercely loyal of whom is Evie. Evie has grown up with Aggs and, excepting her mum and brother, understands her better than anybody. Evie was in their first school play together when Aggs could still walk, and she has memories of what her friend has lost over the years.

I thank the universe for the endlessly kind people in Aggie's world and mine. Those closest to her are all silently hoping that the gene therapy trial she's slated to be on with the new biotech company will take place according to its planned schedule and not be unnecessarily held up by red tape. All I wish for her is the best of health, as ultimately there's nothing more important in life. She is my inspiration, as is her brother.

In the summer of 2024, an uplifting video accumulated more than 60 million views on various social media platforms. It seemed to be on everyone's tablets and phones around the world for weeks.

It's a summer's day outside Horse Guards Parade, as a soldier of the Household Cavalry sits statue-still on his steed, surrounded by hundreds of tourists in a babel of offscreen noise. As tourists from around the globe relentlessly take their position next to the horse for selfies and portraits, one man patiently waits his turn and then pushes his female companion in a wheelchair beside the horse and soldier. She has glacial blue eyes and a warm smile, her blonde hair swept up from her face in a pony tail. The soldier looks at them out of the corner of his eyes beneath the sight-limiting visor of his heavy brass helmet, then slowly, almost imperceptibly, he inches his horse over to the disabled girl, who is busy soaking up the moment in the sunshine. The man sees it sidling over and smiles, then when the horse's head appears right next to his companion, he strokes its nose calmy while protecting the girl by not moving an inch. Then the girl spots the friendly animal and her face lights up with sheer pleasure and she throws her head back in abandon and laughs. She's beautiful. The boy nods in thanks to the rider, then smiles at the horse before slowly pushing the girl away. The whole thing has taken about 30 seconds.

The reason it went viral so quickly was that in a few seconds it conveyed the essence of compassion, protectiveness, surprise, joy and gratitude, as well as stoicism in the face of disability. Though some online wrongly surmised they were husband and wife, the girl is in fact my daughter Aggie, and the man is my son Finn.

Author's Note

My thanks to you, dear reader, for coming with me on this journey. It's not been an easy one and I have taken you through some of my darkest days, but I hope you've got to know me better for the reading of it, and perhaps some of my mental fortitude techniques might be useful to you. I hope, too, that more than a few of you will now be tempted into the cold water where you will find nothing but goodness and wellbeing. Maybe I'll see you out there.

Richard Waters
Autumn 2024